Learning Supportive Psychotherapy

An Illustrated Guide

Arnold Winston, M.D.

Chairman, Department of Psychiatry and Behavioral Sciences,
Beth Israel Medical Center, New York, New York; Professor and
Vice Chairman, Department of Psychiatry and Behavioral Sciences,
Albert Einstein College of Medicine, Bronx, New York

Richard N. Rosenthal, M.D.

Chairman, Department of Psychiatry and Behavioral Health, St. Luke's-
Roosevelt Hospital Center, New York, New York; Arthur J. Antenucci
Professor of Clinical Psychiatry, Department of Psychiatry, and Senior
Associate Dean, Columbia University College of Physicians and
Surgeons, New York, New York

Henry Pinsker, M.D.

Honorary Attending, Department of Psychiatry and Behavioral Sciences,
Beth Israel Medical Center, New York, New York; Clinical Professor of
Psychiatry (retired), Department of Psychiatry, Mount Sinai School of
Medicine, New York, New York

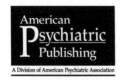

American **Psychiatric** Publishing
A Division of American Psychiatric Association

Washington, DC
London, England

To buy 25–99 copies of this or any other APP title at a 20% discount, please contact Customer Service at appi@psych.org or 800-368-5777. For 100 or more copies of the same title, please e-mail us at bulksales@psych.org for a price quote.

Copyright © 2012 American Psychiatric Association
ALL RIGHTS RESERVED

Manufactured in the United States of America on acid-free paper
15   14   13   12   11   5   4   3   2   1
First Edition

Typeset in Adobe's Berling Roman and Frutiger.

American Psychiatric Publishing,
a Division of American Psychiatric Association
1000 Wilson Boulevard
Arlington, VA 22209–3901
www.appi.org

Library of Congress Cataloging-in-Publication Data
Winston, Arnold, 1935–
   Learning supportive psychotherapy : an illustrated guide / by Arnold Winston, Richard N. Rosenthal, Henry Pinsker.—1st ed.
       p. ; cm. — (Core competencies in psychotherapy)
   Includes bibliographical references and index.
   ISBN 978-1-58562-399-0 (alk. paper)
   1. Supportive psychotherapy. 2. Psychotherapist and patient. I. Rosenthal, Richard N. II. Pinsker, Henry, 1928– III. Title. IV. Series: Core competencies in psychotherapy.
   [DNLM: 1. Psychotherapy—methods. 2. Professional-Patient Relations. 3. Psychotherapeutic Processes. WM 420]
   RC489.S86W56 2011
   616.89'14—dc23

                                                                        2011019043

British Library Cataloguing in Publication Data
A CIP record is available from the British Library.

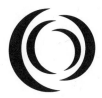

Contents

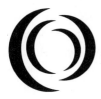

Introduction

We are pleased to present a revised version of our book *Introduction to Supportive Psychotherapy*, first published in 2004. We have made a number of major changes to the book. The most important one is the addition of a DVD with six vignettes illustrating our overall supportive psychotherapy approach and the use of various techniques associated with this modality. The six vignettes also are included in the book.

The chapter on the concept of supportive psychotherapy (Chapter 1) has been completely rewritten, with emphasis on overcoming the confusion of terms that has stemmed from a historical approach focused on the evolutionary development of supportive psychotherapy. We try to make clear that while supportive and expressive therapies are taught as contrasting approaches, in the clinical setting supportive and expressive elements are invariably integrated. Descriptions of treatment tactics have been revised so that material is presented in sequences we have found to be most helpful to beginning therapists. The chapter on general framework (Chapter 5) has been expanded with new illustrations; and in the chapter on applicability to special populations (Chapter 8), we present new research on the effects of supportive psychotherapy in personality disorders, as well as an enhanced clinical vignette that is also included on the DVD. In addition, the chapter on the therapeutic relationship (Chapter 6) contains an expanded clinical vignette that also can be found on the DVD. Chapter 9, on evaluating competence and outcome research, has been updated as well.

When *Introduction to Supportive Psychotherapy* was first published, the Residency Review Committee for Psychiatry had mandated that all psychiatry residents achieve competence in five types of psychotherapy. In 2007, this requirement was changed to three types of psychotherapy: supportive, psychodynamic, and cognitive-behavioral psychotherapies (Accreditation Council for Graduate Medical Education 2007). In this book, we outline a systematic approach to one of these therapies: supportive psychotherapy.

This book is written for beginning therapists who need to learn the fundamentals of psychotherapy, and in particular, to learn how to talk with psychotherapy patients. All practitioners search for effective ways to treat patients. We believe that the beginning resident attempting to practice supportive psychotherapy needs clear guidelines for the conduct and progression of psychotherapy from beginning to end. Accordingly, we have attempted to present straightforward guidelines to help the beginner in four major areas:

- Maintaining a positive therapeutic alliance
- Understanding and formulating patients' problems
- Setting realistic treatment goals
- Knowing what to say to patients (technique)

After introducing the concept of supportive psychotherapy, we present the basic principles of this treatment approach and the position of supportive psychotherapy on a continuum from supportive to expressive psychotherapy, on the basis of the extent and level of a patient's psychopathology. We describe supportive psychotherapy interventions available to the therapist, how to perform a thorough patient evaluation and case formulation, and the process of setting realistic goals with the patient.

The general framework of supportive psychotherapy—including indications, phases of treatment, initiation and termination of sessions, and professional boundaries—are outlined. We include therapeutic relationship issues (transference, countertransference, therapeutic alliance) and self-disclosure guidelines.

We discuss crisis intervention, which uses many supportive psychotherapy approaches, and the applicability of supportive psychotherapy to special populations, including patients with chronic mental illness, substance abuse, and comorbid conditions. We conclude the book with a discussion of how to determine whether a psychiatry resident has achieved competence in supportive psychotherapy and with a presentation of the evidence for the efficacy of supportive psychotherapy, containing a summary of a number of outcome trials.

Arnold Winston, M.D.
Richard N. Rosenthal, M.D.
Henry Pinsker, M.D.

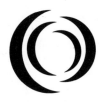

Acknowledgments

We are indebted to a number of colleagues for their help in supplying material for this book and help during its writing. We owe particular thanks to Mimi Lee for her help in preparing the manuscript. Beverly Winston provided important feedback on each of the chapters.

Residents at Beth Israel Medical Center and St. Luke's-Roosevelt Hospital Center were recruited as patients and therapists for the psychotherapy DVD. We are grateful for their efforts in production of the DVD. The following residents participated from Beth Israel Medical Center: Caroline Blackman, M.D., Nivea Calico, M.D., David Edgcomb, M.D., and Glenn Occhiogrosso, M.D. The following residents participated from St. Luke's-Roosevelt Hospital Center: Justin Capote, M.D., Nonso Ekene Enekwechi, M.D., Adrienne Mishkin, M.D., and Vinod Pachagiri Suresh, M.D.

We wish to acknowledge the importance of the Beth Israel Brief Psychotherapy Research Program in providing the milieu for the writing of this book, and our appreciation of our colleagues from this program, especially John Christopher Muran, Jeremy Safran, and Lisa Wallner Samstag. Finally, we are grateful to the Supportive Psychotherapy Study Group, including Victor Goldin, Esther Goldman, David Hellerstein, David Janeway, Steve Klee, Lee Shomstein, Fran Silverman, Jeffrey Solgan, Adam Wilensky, and Philip Yanowitch, for help in developing many of the ideas contained in this book.

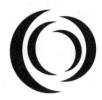

DVD Contents

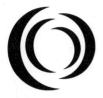

The Concept of Supportive Psychotherapy

Origins

The concept of supportive psychotherapy was developed early in the twentieth century to characterize a treatment approach with objectives more limited than the objectives of psychoanalysis. The objectives of supportive treatment, as initially defined, were not to change a patient's personality, but rather to help a patient cope with symptoms, to prevent relapse of serious mental illness, or to help a relatively healthy person deal with a transient problem. In more recent years, the domain of supportive psychotherapy has become larger, reflecting changes in the definition—and even more so, in the practice—of psychotherapy. Although customarily explained in terms of its origins in psychoanalysis, supportive psychotherapy is a treatment approach that shares tactics and objectives with the medical management that is familiar to physicians who are entering the specialty of psychiatry.

In the early years of the twentieth century, psychoanalysis was essentially the only formal psychological treatment within medicine. Treatment that did not conform to the tenets of psychoanalysis was denigrated as *suggestion*, an approach that had been used with occasional success as a treatment for hysteria, the object of Freud's earliest attention. As well-trained therapists increased their use of supportive approaches and decreased their use of analytic approaches, supportive psychotherapy, now defined more broadly, became the treatment provided to "the vast majority of patients seen in psychiatric clinics and mental health centers" (Werman 1984, p. ix), and suggestion was abandoned as a modality of treatment.

Terminology Dissonance

Douglas (2008) observed as we did in 1986 (Winston et al. 1986) that different authors have proposed different definitions of supportive psychotherapy and that there are differences of opinion about whether supportive psychotherapy is or is not a psychodynamic therapy and whether it is or is not a distinctive form of therapy. The problem of definition is compounded, as we explain in this section, by the coexistence of two incompatible definitions of psychodynamic therapy.

Psychoanalysis and psychotherapy were originally developed as treatments for *neurosis,* which had been the principal concern of office-based (i.e., nonhospital) psychiatrists. Neurosis was conceptualized as an unconscious attempt to solve a psychological conflict. Psychoanalytic thinkers who formulated theories about the causes of symptoms and personality problems ultimately created a general theory of mental organization and behavior that is generally referred to as *psychodynamic theory.* Many concepts of psychodynamic theories have become so widely disseminated that they are now accepted by much of the educated public in the Western world as established truth about mental life.

As psychotherapy became more widely accepted, therapists applied the techniques to a broad range of problems that were outside the scope of the earliest psychotherapy and not adequately explained by the theories associated with it. Furthermore, because of practical considerations, which included payment, the course of treatment often consisted of a small number of visits, with the objective limited to relief of the presenting problem. Therapists found it necessary to be more interactive and responsive with patients. Flexible response to clinical reality called for more general use of supportive approaches, although some therapists feared that they were diluting the "real" psychotherapy by not adhering to its rules. In fact, they were applying a different psychotherapy.

Therapy that was not psychoanalysis but instead was based on theories developed by psychoanalysts became known as *psychodynamic psychotherapy.* At various times it has been called psychoanalytically oriented psychotherapy, intensive psychotherapy, uncovering psychotherapy, change-oriented psychotherapy, insight-directed psychotherapy, or—the term we employ—expressive psychotherapy (not to be confused with dance therapy, art therapy, and so forth, which have also been designated as "expressive"). Between 1950 and 1970, psychodynamic psychotherapy became the most widely practiced psychological treatment approach in the United States. It was taught as the embodiment of theories of personality development, with the objectives of reversing the primary disease process or restructuring the personality (Ursano and Silberman 1999). In the psychotherapy literature, *personality change* is invariably assumed to be the objective. Psychiatrists who work in clinics, however, are responsible for many patients for whom the objective is stability, not change. The inconsistency of definition stems from the fact that some writers use the term *psychodynamic psychotherapy* broadly to describe any therapy in which the therapist's *understanding* of mental life is based on theories developed by psychoanalytic writers, whereas other authors use the term narrowly to describe only therapies that employ the essential *techniques* of expressive therapy.

Definitions of supportive psychotherapy have been organized around four themes:

1. What the therapist hopes to achieve (objectives)—for example, to maintain or improve the patient's self-esteem, to minimize or prevent recurrence of symptoms, and to maximize the patient's adaptive capacities (Pinsker et al. 1991).
2. What the patient wants to achieve (goals)—for example, to maintain or reestablish his or her best possible level of functioning given the limitations of his or her personality, native ability, and life circumstances (Ursano and Silberman 1999).
3. What the therapist does (technique)—for example, encouragement, reassurance, education, and advice.
4. What it is not—an exposition of elements of expressive therapy that have been subtracted (Dewald 1964, 1971).

In addressing the question of where supportive psychotherapy fits among the many models of psychotherapy, Rockland (1989) proposed the acronym POST to signify "psychodynamically oriented supportive therapy," explaining that all psychotherapies involve both supportive and exploratory interventions, and that therapy should be "based on as complete an understanding as possible of the patient's core conflicts, characteristic defensive maneuvers, ego functions, superego organization, and object relations" (p. 7). Although Rockland's acronym has not caught on, his thinking reflects the views of most who have written about supportive psychotherapy in the past 25 years. On the other hand, as described by Mellman and Beresin (2003), the Psychiatry Residency Review Committee stipulated that beginning in 2001, residents must be competent in dynamic psychotherapy and supportive psychotherapy—defining them as distinct modalities. By examining some key concepts of psychodynamic psychotherapy as enumerated by Gabbard (2010, pp. 4–18), we can understand the inconsistent use of the term.

In Gabbard's (2010, p. 4) definition, three elements pertain to the therapist's understanding of the patient:

- Much of mental life is unconscious.
- Childhood experiences in concert with genetic factors shape the adult.
- Symptoms and behaviors serve multiple functions and are determined by complex and often unconscious forces.

Those who describe themselves as psychodynamically oriented practitioners of supportive psychotherapy accept and use these elements.

The next three elements pertain to the therapist's actions, or to the conduct of the treatment:

- The patient's transference to the therapist is a primary source of understanding.
- The therapist's countertransference provides valuable understanding about what the patient induces in others.
- The patient's resistance to the therapy process is a major focus of the therapy.

The therapist conducting supportive psychotherapy is aware of these phenomena but makes use of them only to the extent necessary. In the context of supportive psychotherapy, the term *resistance* may be used to describe the patient's clinging to familiar patterns, with no implications about unconscious process.

The final element describes the objective, or what the therapist hopes to accomplish:

- The goal is to assist the patient in achieving a sense of authenticity and uniqueness.

The formal objectives of supportive psychotherapy are limited to symptom relief and better adaptation.

The "psychodynamically oriented" therapist understands the patient in terms of the first three of Gabbard's (2010) points, but does not conduct treatment in the manner described in the next three points. Also, although the therapist would be pleased to achieve the outcome described in the last point, it would not be the objective.

Novalis et al. (1993, p. 5) observed, "Virtually all of the several hundred psychotherapies are based upon a concept or theory of mind. Supportive psychotherapy...is not dependent upon any specific overriding concept or theory, but utilizes the rich work done by many theorists in understanding how people change as this work is confirmed empirically."

The early characterization of supportive psychotherapy as a limited approach was based on its deviation from classical theory. Although the rationale and techniques of today's supportive psychotherapy can be explained in terms of theory, the techniques were not derived from theory, but rather were developed from work with patients.

Psychodynamic Therapy Spectrum

In his textbook on dynamic psychotherapy, Dewald (1971) explained the contrast between supportive psychotherapy and insight-directed therapy (i.e., expressive therapy, in our terminology), observing that a patient's treatment usually falls someplace between these two ends of the psychotherapeutic spectrum (see Figure 1–1). He described supportive psychotherapy as generally aimed at symptom relief and overt behavior change, without emphasis on modifying personality or resolving unconscious conflict. He wrote, "The majority of people with psychiatric illness, social deviancy, marital disturbances, character problems, acute or chronic psychosis, etc., are not suitable candidates for a formal attempt at insight-directed psychotherapy. Instead they are more suitably and expeditiously treated by a dynamically oriented supportive approach" (p. 114).

The term *expressive therapy* is a collective term for a variety of approaches that seek personality change through analysis of the relationship between therapist and patient and through the acquisition of insight about previously unrecognized feelings, thoughts, needs, and conflicts, following which the patient must attempt to consciously resolve and better integrate such conflicts. We prefer using the term "expressive therapy" in order to avoid using the word *psychodynamic* with two different meanings.

As Dewald (1964) noted, "The ends of the continuum can be clearly distinguished from each other in regards to the theory of psychotherapy, and to the technique which evolves logically from this theory. In the center of the continuum these differences are less discrete and less clearly demarcated. The treatment of most patients involves both supportive and expressive elements, which must be used in a coherent, integrated fashion" (p. 97).

To emphasize that the treatment of each patient involves both supportive and expressive elements, some form of a linear representation of this continuum has been presented by a number of authors (Figure 1–1). At one end, the frequency of supportive interventions is high and the frequency of exploratory intervention is low. At the other end, the frequency of supportive interventions is low. The supportive and expressive *stances,* or points of view, are very different. The most supportive stance involves guidance, whereas the most expressive involves discovery. Luborsky and Mark (1991, p. 110) described expressive therapies as "techniques aimed at facilitating the patient's expressions about problems and conflicts and their understanding." The supportive position may encourage use of a defense; the expressive position may seek to discover the roots of the defense and hope that its use will end. Even though treatment invariably entails both supportive and expressive elements, the therapist's basic stance, at a single point in treatment of a patient, must be primarily one or the other. When the stance is expressive, the therapist follows the dictum to "be as expressive as you can be, and as supportive as you have to be" (Wallerstein 1986, p. 688). When the stance is supportive, the therapist follows Wachtel's (1993) advice: "Be as supportive as you can be so that you can be as expressive as you will need to be" (p. 155). This distinction is critical.

The graphic representation in Figure 1–1 must not be thought of as indicating that the patient population is distributed on a bell-shaped curve. Essentially, when we describe the conceptual basis of therapy, supportive-expressive psychotherapy and expressive-supportive psychotherapy meet at the center of the visual representation; when we describe the universe of patients, we believe that supportive-expressive psychotherapy is what most practitioners are doing most of the time with most of their patients. If asked what they are doing, they will respond "psychotherapy," or "supportive psychotherapy," or "psychoanalytically oriented psychotherapy," or "psychodynamic psychotherapy," or perhaps, facetiously, "general American psychotherapy." It is also important to note that the world of psychotherapy is no longer limited to approaches based on psychodynamic formulations. Supportive interventions may be used productively in the conduct of cognitive-behavioral therapy, for example, without raising significant theoretical or practical problems.

If the treatment of each patient involves both supportive and expressive elements, why are the elements taught separately? As Rockland (1989) pointed out, "Because of their very significant differences, supportive and exploratory psychotherapies do constitute separate treatments, sufficiently discrepant in major ways to deserve clear differentiation and separation" (p. 20). Supportive psychotherapy, expressive

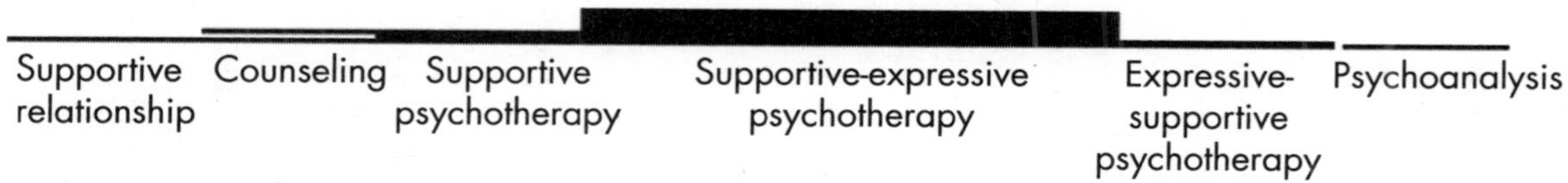

Figure 1–1. Supportive-expressive continuum.

therapy, cognitive-behavioral therapy, family therapy, and group therapy, among others, are all taught by different specialists because there is a lot to know about each of them. It is important to understand, as McWilliams (2004, p. 3) pointed out, that the various features of psychotherapeutic approaches should be compared to a light with a dimmer, not a light controlled by an on/off switch. As in all areas of education, it is the task of the student to integrate all that he or she has been offered. Although in this text we focus on a simple model of expressive psychotherapy in our explanation of the origin of supportive psychotherapy, we appreciate that many, many approaches to therapy have been given names; each approach emphasizes an element of treatment, personality development, or symptom formation that is thought to be novel or especially significant. As Winston and Winston (2002) said, "Although developmental, conflict, and cognitive-behavioral theory are described separately to maintain clarity, these various models come together to inform the psychotherapy approach for a given patient" (p. 13); and "Therapists... should be able to transition from one approach to another. Such transitioning involves combining various interventions from different psychotherapy traditions into a cohesive therapy" (p. 264).

Fonagy and Target (2009) present a summary of "assumptions of modern psychodynamic therapy":

1. Assumption of psychological causation
2. Assumption of limitations of consciousness and the influence of unconscious mental states
3. Assumption of internal representations of interpersonal relationships
4. Assumption of ubiquity of psychological conflict
5. Assumption of psychic defenses
6. Assumption of complex meaning
7. Assumption of emphasis on the therapeutic relationship
8. Assumption of the validity of a developmental perspective

A therapist who accepts these assumptions is a psychodynamically oriented therapist. Dipping into this body of assumptions enriches the expressive component of supportive-expressive psychotherapy.

Definitions

The term *supportive therapy* is frequently used in nonpsychiatric studies to denote the designation for an approach that involves expression of interest, attention to concrete services, encouragement, and optimism. This is a supportive *relationship* or supportive *contact*, but not supportive *psy-*

chotherapy. Supportive psychotherapy is based on diagnostic evaluation; the therapist's actions are deliberate and designed to achieve specified objectives. Supportive relationships with family, friends, coworkers, clergy, and others may indeed be useful and sustaining, but in our opinion should not be called "therapy." We note, too, that the boundary between counseling and psychotherapy is not clear. The professional relationship is unique. It exists solely to meet the needs of the patient (or client). The therapist's gratification must come from doing the job well, rather than from the patient's expressions of gratitude or from using the patient as an audience. In everyday life, there are many motivations for being supportive. In the professional supportive relationship, the motivation must be to meet the patient's needs.

In psychiatric literature, the terms *supportive therapy* and *supportive psychotherapy* have been used interchangeably. This is unfortunate, because the nonspecific support provided to patients who have medical or surgical problems is also characterized as "supportive therapy," in this case referring to efforts that make the patient more comfortable but do not remediate the underlying problem. We will always use the long form—*supportive psychotherapy*—to emphasize that we are writing about a professional service that is provided in a mental health context by a person trained in mental health theory and practices.

We define *supportive psychotherapy* as a dyadic treatment that uses direct measures 1) to ameliorate symptoms and 2) to maintain, restore, or improve self-esteem, ego function, and adaptive skills. To the extent necessary to accomplish these objectives, treatment may examine relationships, real or transferential, and both past and current patterns of emotional response or behavior.

- *Self-esteem* involves the patient's sense of efficacy, confidence, hope, and self-regard.
- *Ego functions* include relation to reality, thinking, defense formation, regulation of affect, synthetic function, and others as enumerated by Beres (1956, pp. 164–235), Bellak (1958, pp. 1–40), and other authors. Ego functions could alternatively be called "psychological functions," because they are addressed by behavior therapists and cognitive therapists whose formulations do not include the ego as a component of a mental apparatus. Ego functions are often categorized as "psychic structure." As cognitive functions are increasingly understood in physical and physiological terms, psychological terminology may be eclipsed, but at present, it still appears useful in the clinical setting.
- *Adaptive skills* are actions associated with effective functioning. The boundary between ego functions and adaptive skills is not sharply de-

fined. The patient's assessment of events is an ego function; the action taken in response to the assessment is an adaptive skill.

We have explained that supportive and expressive therapies are quite different, and we have explained how the treatment of an individual patient is likely to involve elements of both. In practice, the term *supportive psychotherapy*, according to the definition we have offered, describes what is usually identified on the continuum as supportive-expressive psychotherapy. When we teach or prescribe "psychodynamic therapy," we usually mean expressive-supportive psychotherapy. Most psychotherapists in the United States are guided by psychodynamic principles, but it is possible to address self-esteem issues, ego-function problems, and adaptive skills without accepting psychodynamic principles.

Case Illustrations

In the following three examples, the therapists' approaches represent different points along the supportive-expressive continuum.

Juan is a 55-year-old man who attended school for 6 years in his native Latin American country. In the United States, he had various unskilled jobs. He was married for several years but was divorced by his wife when he became involved with drugs. Since a 2-year prison stay 20 years ago, he has been drug-free but has had increased difficulty obtaining work because of his record. He now has several medical problems; he keeps his clinic appointments and follows prescribed treatment. He has been seen once a month in the psychiatric clinic for over a year by a resident who monitors antidepressant medication. Juan attends a day program for medical patients but has been threatened with expulsion because he is quick to show anger and lash out if he feels that someone is pushing him aside at lunchtime or is taking a seat that he wished to occupy. The day program and his clinic visits are his only structured activity. The treating resident discusses with Juan the recommendations of the other physicians and talks about the effects of medications to be sure that Juan will tell the other physicians about any problems. The resident responds empathically to Juan's description of loneliness and praises him for his success at maintaining sobriety. The resident is satisfied that Juan's angry responses are not associated with delusional thinking, but the resident has been unable to involve Juan in scrutinizing the reason for his responses or offering anything but the most superficial justifications for his actions. Juan does, however, accept the suggestion that he should always seek help from a staff member if he is angered by other participants in the day program. *(This is an entirely supportive approach, involving encouragement, praise, and advice about adaptive skills. Success will be measured by the patient's continued acceptance of medical treatment, antidepressant medication, and ability to control his temper.)*

Carlos has the same problems as Juan (above) but has a greater ability to think about his internal life. He says that if someone gets ahead of him, he feels that this person is putting him down and mocking him. After all, Carlos says, he was brought up this way. When he did not stand up for himself, his father would become very angry and might punish him, and no one in his community would have considered his father to be wrong. The therapist explains that people brought up by these standards are often too quick to defend themselves from what appears to be an affront, and the patient agrees that this makes sense. *(The therapy in this case is supportive-expressive because it involves assumptions about mental life. The therapist seeks to help the patient begin to understand problem-causing behavior in terms of attitudes about which he had been unaware.)*

George was aware of having an "anger problem" and became very irritable when his therapist asked, as he had at previous sessions, whether George had been involved in any conflicts since the last visit. The patient responded sullenly and then told the therapist that the medication he had been taking for several months was causing too many side effects and wasn't helping at all. The therapist suggested that maybe being asked about possible failures of self-control reminded George of his childhood experience of being scolded by his father. George said he hadn't thought of it, but it might be true. *(Suspecting that the patient's anger might be of transferential origin, the therapist suggests a link between past and present relationships—an expressive element. This therapy may be described as located at the midpoint of the supportive-expressive spectrum.)*

Education

Although supportive psychotherapy is the most widely practiced form of psychodynamically oriented psychotherapy, teaching supportive psychotherapy poses its challenges. Supportive psychotherapy is not based on an appealing theory, and it does not offer solutions to intractable clinical problems; the field has no conferences, no stars, and relatively few books. Education of psychotherapists throughout much of the twentieth century was based primarily on principles developed by psychoanalysts. For example, in a short text for beginners, Balsam and Balsam (1984) wrote, "The psychotherapist's central task is learning to understand the patient.... The focus of the exploration is on understanding the emotional experience of the patient" (p. 1). Treatment techniques that had specific rationales in psychoanalysis were presented as universal techniques required for *all* psychotherapy. For example, if the patient stopped talking, the therapist was advised to wait for him or her to continue or to ask what he or she was thinking. The therapist was advised to avoid direct answers to questions (Colby 1951, pp. 55–56). In short, a treatment intended "to relieve the patient of distressing neurotic symptoms or discordant personality characteristics" (Colby 1951, p. 3) was being taught. However, novice therapists might be assigned patients who are inarticulate or poorly educated or patients who have intractable social problems or severe behavioral problems. Many patients are seen only once or twice a month, and the therapist recognizes the possibility that patients might drop out after a few visits. Therefore, the ideal model that had been taught provided no guidance about how to work with these patients. Some trainees, with innate interpersonal skills and empathy, were effective from the start. Most new clinicians, as they matured in practice, figured out how to be effective, although many thought of themselves as deviating from proper form. Those who became clinical supervisors taught by example. In contrast, psychotherapists who failed to discover how to conduct supportive psychotherapy provided their patients an irrational, unintegrated mixture of expressive assumptions and supportive tactics. As Werman (1984) observed, "the patient and therapist may continue their meetings for an inordinately long time under the illusion that ongoing insight-oriented psychotherapy is actually taking place, when in fact patient and therapist are merely playing a charade" (p. 12).

Patients who are the most mentally intact are suitable for treatment that is primarily expressive, but the fact that a patient has the resources and psychological characteristics that are necessary for the conduct of expressive therapy does not mean that expressive therapy is indicated. Although a blend that provides more support than needed may be effective, it may deprive the patient of an opportunity to make more impressive changes in his or her life. However, as Hellerstein et al. (1994) pointed out, a strong case can be made for employing the supportive (i.e., supportive-expressive) model for most patients, shifting to more expressive measures only to the extent required. In all cases, treatment planning must involve consideration of what the patient wants to accomplish.

The fundamental objectives of supportive psychotherapy at the supportive end of the continuum can be achieved by a clinician who is unsophisticated about psychodynamic principles. Beginners who cannot yet attempt expressive psychotherapy may be competent at providing good supportive-expressive treatment. With practice, therapists become aware of how a patient is responding to them, and then of how they are responding to the patient. Empathic connection to patients may develop slowly over the years. Viederman (2008) described a very active approach, in which the clinician asks the patient for memories about earlier times in life that are related to the clinician's observations and interpretations, and communicates to the patient an understanding of the patient's predicament. He wrote, "The consultant enters the patient's world, develops a picture of him, of his experience with people in his life, and communicates this in a language which is familiar to him. This results in a climate that is the essence of a supportive relationship" (p. 352). One of the many satisfactions of being a psychotherapist is that the clinician improves and continues to improve as the decades pass. The experienced, sophisticated therapist can do sophisticated supportive psychotherapy.

Conclusion

Supportive psychotherapy and the expressive psychotherapies have different objectives and utilize different techniques. The treatment of an individual patient whose treatment plan calls for psychodynamically oriented supportive psychotherapy involves both supportive and expressive elements. The clinician must understand both approaches and be able to integrate them.

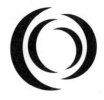

2

Principles and Mode of Action

Underlying Assumptions

Supportive psychotherapy relies on *direct measures*. It is not assumed that improvement will develop as a by-product of insight. A major tenet of Freud's early work in psychoanalysis was that the unconscious conflict that had produced the symptom would become conscious and be worked through, and then the symptom would disappear because it was no longer psychologically necessary. In contrast, supportive psychotherapy addresses conscious problems or conflicts, but not underlying unconscious conflicts and personality distortions (Dewald 1994). Greater self-awareness or insight about the origin of problems is not essential, although it may occur and be productive. Expressive psychotherapies are inherently supportive because of the interest and attention of the therapist, but support is an epiphenomenon in expressive therapy—one that may contribute significantly to the outcome.

In supportive therapy, the *relationship* between patient and therapist is a relationship between two adults with a common purpose. One provides a service that the other needs, similar in most respects to all professional relationships. The professional person, the therapist, owes the patient or client respect, full attention, honesty, and vigorous effort to accomplish the stated purpose by using the knowledge and skills of the profession. Adhering to this discipline is known as staying within boundaries. The interaction may be friendly, but the two individuals do not become friends. The patient may need love, but the therapist does not become a lover. The therapist does not help the sexually naive patient by offering sexual contact. The therapist does not advise the patient how to vote, whom to marry, or how to decorate the home. The therapist does not seek assistance from the patient. If the therapist talks at length, describing his or her own experiences, thoughts, or feelings, the therapist must consider whether it is for the patient's benefit or because the therapist enjoys talking. To use the patient in this manner is exploitation.

When the therapist's stance is expressive, the therapist tries to maintain neutrality and to remain cautious about responses so that the patient's perception of thoughts and feelings about the therapist can be analyzed as projections of feelings associated with important figures in past or present life. This projection is termed *transference*. The expressive stance avoids responses that might encourage the patient to perceive the therapist as a person with opinions, tastes, family, or even personality. It is this technical maneuver that in the past produced an image of the psychotherapist as an individual who parries all questions with evasive answers or by reflecting the question back to the patient.

The degree to which the therapist and patient discuss transference depends on the type of therapy. In expressive therapies, analysis of the transference is a key element of the process of understanding the patient's inner life. Although transference occurs in supportive psychotherapy, as it does in all relationships, it typically is discussed only when manifestations of transference threaten the continuation of therapy. Because in practice most psychotherapy is supportive-expressive, transference is not a taboo subject. In relational therapies, which have been increasingly popular since the 1980s (Fonagy and Target 2009; Greenberg 2001; Mitchell 1988), intense and ongoing examination of the patient-therapist interaction is a major focus of the therapeutic process, and the therapist may disclose much more than would be done in classical treatment. This is not an approach to be undertaken by the novice therapist. Even at the supportive end of the spectrum, it is often useful for a therapist to try to make a patient aware of problems in their real-time interaction.

> Therapist 1: You haven't said you disagree with me, but you have found something wrong with every suggestion I have made. *(A clarification that might encourage patient to be more frank, without examining underlying issues)*
> Therapist 2: Are you aware that whenever I try to focus on steps you might take to manage better in daily life, you go back to talking about what your parents did wrong? *(An observation in the course of supportive-expressive therapy)*

Therapist 3: Are you aware that when I ask you about your father, you talk about problems at work or the world situation? *(Confrontation in the course of expressive-supportive therapy)*

As stated earlier this chapter, the supportive psychotherapy relationship is a relationship between two adults with a common purpose. The therapist encourages the development of positive feelings; if the patient brings up the presence of these positive feelings, the therapist accepts them without attempting to have the patient understand them. The patient's positive feelings about the therapist, even if moderately unrealistic, are useful for maintaining the therapeutic alliance and potentially useful for identification with the therapist (see Chapter 6, "The Therapeutic Relationship," for further discussion of the patient-therapist relationship).

Patient 1: You always have such a clear way of thinking about things. I'm all over the place. You always know what the problem is and what to do about it.
Therapist 1: Thanks. It's easier when you hear a description of a complex issue than when you're in the midst of it.

If negative feelings about the therapist or the therapy are evident, or even suspected, they must be discussed, because negative feelings may threaten or lead to disruption of treatment.

Patient 2: Getting here seems to be more difficult. Things always come up at the last minute. I apologize for being late.
Therapist 2: We could try to change your appointment time if that would help, but I wonder if you're finding it more difficult now because you're having some doubts about continuing.

In expressive psychotherapy, the patient's reaction to events in his or her current life may be discussed as possible (unconscious) expressions of the patient's feelings about the therapist.

Patient: I was on the phone with customer service for half an hour. This really drives me up the wall. It was worse than ever. Those people are incompetent.
Therapist: Last week you were complaining because I hadn't come up with a quick answer for all your problems. Maybe you were especially angry with customer service and saw them as incompetent because you were thinking I was incompetent and you were angry with me.

In supportive psychotherapy, however, events in the therapy may be offered as illustrations or models for everyday life.

Patient: This really drives me up the wall. It was worse than ever. Those people are incompetent.

Therapist: Last week you were complaining because I hadn't come up with a quick answer for all your problems. You were polite, and we were able to discuss it, and you didn't seem to be "up the wall." Maybe you could be as reasonable and controlled when you talk to customer service as you are here with me.

In the course of supportive psychotherapy and supportive-expressive therapy, the therapist gives simple, direct answers to personal questions, within the bounds of information that he or she is willing to share with an acquaintance. Disclosure of information that is ordinarily kept private is often associated with violation of the boundary that must separate the personal from the professional. When the stance is primarily expressive, the therapeutic strategy is based on the assumption that the patient's thoughts about the therapist will reveal evidences of transference.

Conversational Style

Supportive psychotherapy is conducted in a conversational style. Because conversation is the principal form of interaction among adults, readers might wonder why it is necessary for us to say anything about it in this book. When we first wrote about supportive psychotherapy, it was important to convey to the beginner that the therapist's task was not listening silently to a patient who had been instructed to "say whatever comes to mind." Now, the psychiatry resident who listens silently at length usually does so because he or she does not know what to say, or expects the patient to pause at any moment, or hopes that the next sentence will be important and that the patient will soon get to the point. The beginning therapist probably knows that by interrupting a silence too quickly, he or she may never know what is troubling the patient. When the therapeutic stance is supportive, the therapist will not wait long. Faced with a long pause, the expressive therapist thinks, "Is there an indication for me to speak?" In contrast, the supportive therapist thinks, "Is there a reason for me *not* to speak?"

The therapeutic interaction is conversational in style, yet it is not normal conversation. In normal conversation, the speakers alternate: your turn, my turn. You tell me what happened on your way to work this morning, and I tell you what happened to me on the way to work; you talk about your pets, and I talk about my pets. In therapy, the therapist is *responsive*, but it is always the patient's turn.

Physicians who are new to psychotherapy often have had years of practice polishing a style of communication that is not responsive and not supportive. They have mastered the art of obtaining the history by asking questions. When every utterance is a question, the process is interrogation. Miller and Rollnick (1991, p. 66), writing about motivational interviewing, advise that one should not ask more than three questions in a row because doing so implies an interaction between an active expert and a passive patient. To maintain a supportive conversational style, the therapist must be responsive. In the act of responding, the therapist is giving something to the patient. Except for narcissistic individuals who get satisfaction from having an audience, people want to be given something in return for what they give, and this giving, by an intelligent, interested person—the therapist—is gratifying and reassuring.

To maintain a conversational style, the therapist responds both to what the patient volunteers and to the patient's responses to questions.

> Patient: I slept better most of the time.
> Therapist 1: OK.
> Patient: But it's still hard being out of work; I'm just getting by on my unemployment checks.
> Therapist 1: OK.
> Patient: I try to keep busy, like you said.
> Therapist 1: OK.
> Patient: But I still feel bad some of the time.
> Therapist 1: OK. *(This is a dreadful, nongiving, ticlike style of response, not unusual in hospitals.)*

> Patient: I slept better most of the time.
> Therapist 2: I'm glad to hear it. And that's without medication, isn't it?
> Patient: Yes. But it's still hard being out of work; I'm just getting by on my unemployment checks.
> Therapist 2: When you are used to working, unemployment insurance is important, but it doesn't fill your life.
> Patient: I try to keep busy, like you said.
> Therapist 2: Good. What are you doing?
> Patient: I've been cleaning my basement, bit by bit. Not just the floor, but cleaning the old grit from overhead pipes and things like that. It's not really important.
> Therapist 2: It sounds like a project that isn't exciting, but you can see the results of what you have done.
> Patient: But I still feel bad some of the time.
> Therapist 2: I'm sorry to hear it. We have to work on that. *(Therapist's responses, although not profound, indicate interest and concern.)*

The physician who has many patients and little time is tortured by patients who are diffuse and vague. To manage this problem, physicians develop habits of asking leading questions, asking questions that include prompted answers (including multiple-choice lists), or questions that invite yes-no answers.

Therapist 1: Did you leave school because you had to work to help the
family? *(Better question: I'd like to know about your decision to
quit school.)*
Therapist 2: Did your mother think it was a good idea for you to quit
school, or did she object? *(Better question: What did your mother
say about your decision to quit school?)*
Therapist 3: How much do you drink? A little wine with meals? *(Better
question: What is your usual use of alcohol?)*

The open-ended question has the greatest potential for eliciting information. Prompts and suggestions are appropriate when the patient is unable to respond to a broad question. Prompts that elicit a "no" answer or
multiple-choice lists that fail to include a correct alternative may cause
the patient to infer that the therapist does not understand.

The beginner therapist who has overcome the habit of asking questions
is at risk of falling into unproductive agreeableness, always responding to
the patient's most recent words. The therapist asks a question, the patient
gives a partial answer and then moves to another topic, the therapist asks
a question about that, and the process is repeated, with the therapist
never having the opportunity to deal with anything useful. Beginning
therapists are often easily put off because if a patient's answer is not adequate, they go on to another question instead of pursuing an answer to
the initial question. In short, asking too many questions is not good form,
but if a question is asked, it should not be abandoned without an attempt
to get an answer. The therapist who does not attempt to understand the
whole story sends the message that he or she does not really care.

Therapist 1: Do you have any thoughts about any issues or events that
may have led up to your depression last year?
Patient: Nothing. It just happened. It came out of the blue.
Therapist 1: Have you ever felt suicidal? *(Therapist, if curious about
what led to the depression, should have attempted to persist with
that topic even though suicide is also an important issue.)*

Therapist 2: What was happening in your life in the month or so before
the depression began? *(Persisting with a general question that does
not call on patient to make cause-and-effect connections)*
Patient: Nothing special. I went to work. I came home. My husband was
working. The kids were in school. *(Uninformative)*
Therapist 2: Let's take them one at a time. What about work? What were
you doing? What about coworkers? Any problems? Did anyone you
care about leave? Was your assignment changed? Your supervisor?
Advancement? *(By deliberately offering multiple-choice options,
therapist teaches about topics that might be important.)*
Patient: Not really. Everything was routine. *(Uninformative)*
Therapist 2: OK. Tell me about your husband and children at that time.

What was going on? We are looking for things that might have been disturbing but that you might have brushed aside at the time without paying much attention. *(The prodding question is asked in a supportive way. Although suggesting answers to questions was described earlier as bad form, it may be used as a tactic for educating patient about important issues and maintaining focus.)*

Seeking more complete information about what the patient is saying is a demonstration of interest and attention, so it is a supportive act, provided the pursuit of additional information does not take on the quality of attack. The key to obtaining complete information is often the wonderful phrase, "give me an example."

Patient 1: If I get mad at work, I just don't go back.
Therapist 1: Give me an example. What was the incident that got to you?
Patient 1: It was nothing. I was working a counter. A customer was arguing with me.
Therapist 1: So a customer started to argue with you. Let's try and look at what happened. What did the customer say, and what did you say?

Patient 2: I have to do everything. My husband is helpless in the house. I come home from work and I have to get dinner, even though he's been home.
Therapist 2: What do you mean by "helpless"? Does he do any tasks at all?

Patient 3: No, I never get angry. I can't remember ever losing my temper.
Therapist 3: Can you describe some instance in which something displeased you a little?

Maintaining and Improving Self-Esteem

Maintaining or improving self-esteem is a major concern of supportive psychotherapy. One person helps the self-esteem of another person by conveying acceptance, approval, interest, respect, or admiration. The person whose daily life and relationships are lacking or deficient in these qualities may respond to any indication of their presence. The patient who cannot form relationships with others, who is avoided by others, or who perceives (perhaps correctly) that people look at him or her disapprovingly, finds in the therapist a person who is accepting and interested. The therapist's acceptance and respect are unspoken. The therapist communicates interest in the patient by making it evident that he or she remembers their conversations, recalls what the patient has said, and is aware of the patient's likes, dislikes, and attitudes. Acceptance is communicated by avoidance of arguing, denigrating, and criticizing—verbal interactions common to many relationships, including, unfortunately, many contacts between patients and health care providers.

Therapist 1: It doesn't make any sense to get an MRI [magnetic resonance image] just because you forget people's names. *(Argument)*
Therapist 2: What are you trying to say? *(Denigration)*
Therapist 3: Didn't they tell you to take your medication every day? *(Criticism)*

Here are the responses in more congenial language.

Therapist 1: Forgetting names is usually the first defect in memory that normal people experience. If that is the only problem, it's not caused by the sort of thing that shows up on an MRI.
Therapist 2: I don't understand.
Therapist 3: A lot of the effect is lost if you don't take your medication every day. If the dosage is too large, we should discuss it. A smaller dosage might be the answer.

In their efforts to boost or avoid lowering the patient's self-esteem, therapists need to avoid language that is overpowering (directly or by implication) and behavior that may make the patient feel diminished or helpless, such as pomposity, overelaborate speech, or ostentatiousness. The following are some overpowering statements:

Therapist 1: I'm trying to get you to understand…
Therapist 2: I'm going to medicate you.
Therapist 3: It's your imagination.

These are better ways to express the same ideas:

Therapist 1: I hope I'm being clear.
Therapist 2: Let's talk about medication.
Therapist 3: When you hear something that people around you don't hear, it's not imagination; it's an event in your brain that's not triggered by something in the environment.

Questions that begin with the words *why* or *why didn't you* are often experienced as attacks, and they should be avoided (Pinsker 1997). In the course of growing up, most people learn that "Why did you do it?" is not so much a search for information as a rebuke for having committed a certain act. Similarly, "Why didn't you do it?" means "You should have done it." Attack is inimical to self-esteem. Alternatives to *why* questions can be created:

Therapist 1: Can you explain how it was that you did it that way?
Therapist 2: When you dropped out of school, what was the reason?
Therapist 3: Was there something about your behavior that made them think it was necessary to call the police?

Attacking questions are accepted as a matter of course in most relationships, and they are certainly customary in conventional medical practice, so reasonable use of them is not going to destroy the therapy. The objective is to conduct therapy with finesse, thus enhancing the prospects for success. In the same vein, when possible, it is better practice to ask questions in a way that elicits a positive response rather than a negative response. For example, it is better to ask an obese person, "Do you find it difficult to exercise?" than to ask, "Do you exercise?" It is better to ask a general question, when possible, than a narrow question. For example, "What are you serving for dessert?" is a better question than "Are you serving cake?" The therapist should not be a person to whom the patient must too often answer "No." Asking questions that are likely to be answered "no" implies that the therapist does not understand the patient.

The doctor-patient relationship involves a person who has the power to give help and a person who needs help. The doctor should give help in a skillful manner that minimizes the inherent inequality of the transaction and communicates respect for the patient. Respect is good for self-esteem and good for the therapeutic alliance. Giving the patient vague, dismissive explanations conveys lack of respect.

Patient 1: I think this medication is making me sleepy.
Physician 1: It hasn't been a problem for most people. How's your appetite? *(Dismissive)*

Patient 2: I don't feel any better.
Physician 2: Well, you look better. *(If coupled with explanation that depressed people look better before they feel better, this would be fine. As an abrupt response, it is dismissive and argumentative.)*

Even educated, sophisticated patients tend to tolerate disrespectful attitudes of health care providers, because the patients are dependent on them. Patients tend to tolerate disrespectful attitudes and behavior from health care providers because they are dependent on them and cannot risk animosity. The patient may employ the defenses of rationalization or denial to avoid awareness of resentment. For many individuals, the reality of needing care has a negative effect on self-esteem. The health care provider should not rub salt into the wound.

We recommend that therapists discuss with the patient the reason for questions, explain the direction being taken, and ask the patient for agreement about topics to be discussed. We refer to these tactics as "setting the agenda" or "showing the map." For patients, these tactics help to prevent both the anxiety that may be associated with going in unknown directions and the interrogatory atmosphere that reinforces the idea that the patient is in an inferior position.

Defenses

In the supportive approach, defenses are encouraged (supported) when they serve their unconscious purpose—protecting the individual from anxiety or other unpleasant affect. When therapy is primarily expressive, defenses are identified and examined to discover the underlying conflicts that made the defenses necessary. In supportive psychotherapy, defenses are questioned only when they are maladaptive. For example, a patient's denial as a strategy for not thinking about the inevitably fatal outcome of his or her own life is adaptive, whereas a patient's denial that leads to his or her refusal of potentially safe and beneficial treatment is maladaptive. Another example is that a careful, compulsive style is useful for a medical student, but compulsive behavior that interferes with work or relationships is maladaptive. In expressive psychotherapy, passive-aggressive behavior might be explored as an indicator of unconscious hostility and a need to control others; in supportive psychotherapy, the same behavior might be accepted as adaptive. When dealing with defenses, the situation is fluid—a therapist may support one defense and question another. Also, a therapist might recognize and not question a defense early in treatment but question it later in treatment.

In maintaining the supportive stance in the therapist-patient relationship, the therapist should consider it permissible and desirable to explore the meaning of the patient's actions and thoughts. Whether the therapist supports, ignores, or questions a statement that appears to reflect a defensive position depends on the current situation, including the context of the patient-therapist conversation (e.g., the therapist must consider whether to interrupt the patient to raise a question or to go along with the patient's flow). The following are examples of different responses:

> Patient: I hated being in the hospital. Every day someone would be acting up, and they'd jump on him with a needle. I was glad I wasn't that bad off.
> Therapist 1: Yeah. *(Accepts the defense without comment)*
> Therapist 2: Maybe you were afraid on some level that it could happen to you. A lot of people equate mental illness with being out of control, so if they find themselves in a hospital because they have a mental illness, they are afraid they may be in danger of being out of control. *(Proposes an explanation for the defense, using the technique of "normalization" to lessen the impact)*
> Therapist 3: Yes. Your condition was quite different. Severe depression is one thing; a psychotic episode is another. That wouldn't happen to you. *(Encourages the defense)*

When does the therapist need to be expressive? Whenever the basic supportive techniques do not appear to be enough to accomplish the patient's goals and if it appears that the patient's life can be improved by use of expressive techniques. The expressive techniques can be used without altering the supportive stance. As stated in Chapter 1, "The Concept of Supportive Psychotherapy," the therapist must know whether his or her basic stance with a patient is supportive or expressive—the therapist cannot maintain both transference-encouraging neutrality and a real relationship at the same time.

Psychodynamic Assumptions

Many physicians begin psychiatric training without having had exposure to psychodynamics or any form of psychotherapy. Some trainees are from countries where psychodynamic thinking has not been widely disseminated. They may not know what to talk about with a patient after completing the history, hoping that in some way, if the patient talks about his or her past and feelings, improvement will occur. Therefore, for the absolute beginner (and no one else), we offer a few words about psychodynamics.

Psychodynamics is the interaction between conscious and unconscious elements of mental life. It is an explanation of the meaning of behavior. One of the tasks of psychotherapy is to create order out of symptoms and dysfunctions. To accomplish this task, the patient and therapist join in developing a history or narrative in which these symptoms and dysfunctions make sense. Cause-and-effect connections are established. Different schools of psychodynamic thinking may derive different explanations at times. The process of making a comprehensible story may be what matters most.

Case Illustrations

The following are a few examples of psychodynamic formulations.

David, a man who is ordinarily self-sufficient and cheerful, becomes demanding and uncooperative when hospitalized following a heart attack, although he has been reassured that his prognosis is very good. A psychodynamic hypothesis might be that the passive, somewhat helpless role of hospital patient is anxiety provoking, and David is attempting to compensate by assuming an overbearing attitude. Because he is unaware that the enforced passivity is behind his unusual behavior, his behavior is considered to be unconscious.

After being criticized by his parents for watching television all night, Mark, a patient with schizophrenia, becomes angry with his parents and stops taking his antipsychotic medication. According to his chart, he has been educated about taking the medication and has verbalized under-standing. He is not aware that "forgetting" to take his medication may be psychologically motivated defiance.

Home for Thanksgiving during his first year of college, Zach, a healthy teenager, provokes a big argument the day before he leaves home, with the consequence that when he leaves, he is angry. He is not aware that part (not all) of him would like to stay home and be dependent. By going away angry, he is protected from the sadness that is part of his departure.

Susan comes regularly for clinic visits, each time giving a detailed account of how other people abuse her. After many attempts to get Susan to ex-amine her role in causing or maintaining at least some of her troubles, the therapist suggests that therapy is unproductive and should be discontin-ued because it will be seen as poor utilization of resources. A psychody-namic hypothesis might be that because repeating familiar patterns is an anxiety-reducing element of human behavior, Susan may be setting up a situation in which she will be rejected, thus confirming her expectations about relationships with people.

Unrecognized Emotions

An assumption of psychodynamically oriented therapies is that unrecog-nized emotions are often responsible for current unpleasant feelings or maladaptive behavior. At times, simply becoming aware of the emotions may provide relief. More often, the discovery of the feeling must be fol-lowed by conscious decisions about more effective methods of coping—this is the adaptive skills focus of supportive psychotherapy. In the past, many patients' symptoms were related to what they perceived as unac-ceptable sexual feelings—a problem that is less common today. Unrecog-nized anger is a frequently seen problem ("getting the anger out" was once proposed as a simple, curative tactic but is now recognized as counter-productive). Other often-hidden feelings might be grief that was not ex-perienced at the time of an important loss, or guilt or hopelessness—or a wish to be admired or to be obeyed. Some individuals are scarcely aware of any feelings at all (the term *alexithymia* has been used to describe them). For them, an important objective is to recognize, acknowledge, identify, and label emotions (Misch 2000). The general task is to incor-porate awareness of feelings into the fabric of memories and current life.

The beginner therapist often asks, "How did it feel?" or "How does it feel?" in response to almost anything the patient says, with no intent or plan about what to do with the answer. However, if the therapist and pa-tient are working on the problem of unrecognized feelings, the patient's feelings connected to events in the past should be explored. They should be explored if the therapist and patient are examining coping strategies, or if the therapist is seeking opportunities to expand his or her empathic understanding. Often, with respect to a current feeling, the question to discuss must be "What is going to be done about it?" The question "What did you think?" is as useful as "What did you feel?" because it pertains to thought process, reality testing, or adaptive skills. In short, the person who knows only thoughts and does not know feelings needs to feel more, whereas the person who feels too much needs to think and evaluate more. Usually, however, therapeutic dialogue involves both feelings and thoughts. Jumping to adaptive solutions without understanding the patient's emotional response is as wrong as ignoring adaptive strategies.

The question "How did you feel?" is pertinent when it initiates discussion of how the patient dealt with the feeling, or if there was no feeling, discussion of the possibility that this lack of feeling is of itself an important finding.

> Patient: I asked the guy next door to go to the mall with me, but he said he didn't have time. He doesn't have any more to do than I do.
> Therapist: How did you feel about that?
> Patient: It's all right. He doesn't have to. *(Evasive, denying emotional response)*
> Therapist: You're right. He doesn't have to. That's a correct analysis. *(Praise)* But you're offering an analysis when I asked about your feelings. *(Confrontation; implied question)*
> Patient: I didn't feel anything.
> Therapist: You describe a situation in which most people would feel disappointment or anger. That reaction won't control the other person, but it's important to know what your feelings are because when you don't, you can't make good decisions about things that affect you. *(Teaching, normalizing)*

Maladaptive Behaviors

Another tenet of psychodynamically oriented therapy is that people often follow patterns of behavior that were appropriate when established but now have become maladaptive. For example, during adolescence, when it is important to reduce emotional dependency on parents, many people assume a belligerent or defiant style. This attitude may be appropriate at age 16 but become a continual source of trouble if it persists at age 26, 46, or 66. Some people, once they see that they are clinging to a pattern of behavior that is familiar and understandable but no longer useful, are able, with determined effort, to change their habitual responses. Cognitive-behavioral therapy focuses on the assumptions associated with patterns of thought and provides tactics for overcoming these assumptions.

Although cognitive and psychodynamic approaches are usually taught separately, tactics of both approaches are integrated in everyday treatment.

The search for patterns that may explain symptoms or maladaptive behavior is the expressive component of supportive-expressive psychotherapy. Once the therapist is past the history-eliciting phase of treatment, he or she is concerned first about feelings and assumptions that are present but unexpressed, then about feelings and assumptions that are lightly concealed, and later about feelings and assumptions that have been truly hidden. A long-familiar analogy is that psychotherapy is like peeling an onion.

Psychogenetics and Early Life Experiences

Psychodynamic explanations tell about the interplay of factors in current life; they do not explain the origins of the forces, emotions, or assumptions that affect behavior. *Psychogenetics* is the search for these origins. When a therapist says that a man who seeks to have sexual relationships with as many women as possible has a "Don Juan syndrome," the therapist is giving a diagnosis (a syndrome diagnosis, not a DSM diagnosis). When the therapist says that the patient acts this way to compensate for insecurity about his masculinity, the therapist is making a psychodynamic hypothesis. When the therapist says that the patient is insecure because he was afraid of his overbearing father, the therapist is proposing a genetic hypothesis. In the case of a woman in her late 30s who is readily able to form relationships but always ends them by discovering faults in her partner and shifting from loving behavior to quarreling, a psychodynamic possibility is that she is unconsciously fearful of closeness or intimacy.

The interpersonal and emotional experiences of early life are important in the development of the individual and his or her problems. Creating a meaningful autobiography is in itself useful, because during the process, what may have appeared to be random events become connected into a meaningful story.

The problem for the beginning therapist is that some patients talk endlessly about their terrible childhoods, emphasizing how they suffered various forms of maltreatment. The inexperienced therapist may feel hopeful that something good will come of allowing the ongoing talk by a patient who is avoiding any discussion about changing his or her patterns or manner of relating to people. Indeed, ventilation can be a legitimate supportive tactic that is useful when the patient has been unable to put painful experiences into words, perhaps because he or she has been afraid to do so or because no one has been available to listen and understand. Recounting the same story also may be adaptive when the patient's goal is limited to relapse prevention and the therapist's objective is to preserve the status quo; however, such retelling is maladaptive when the goal is to improve the patient's life.

Mode of Action

Attempts to achieve the supportive psychotherapy objectives of improved ego function and adaptive skills involve teaching, encouragement, exhortation, modeling, and anticipatory guidance. People in general, not only patients, respond to teaching and instruction if they want to learn, if they want to improve their lot, and if they trust the teacher. They may cooperate with the teacher to please him or her. Such cooperation has been described in psychoanalytic writing as a "transference cure." The Menninger psychotherapy research project found that changes that appeared to come about for this reason proved stable and durable (Wallerstein 1989). Sometimes, advice or instruction from another person, especially an authority figure, is a catalyst, allowing the patient to accomplish change that he or she had already formulated.

Competing claims of the many approaches to psychotherapy produced extensive research aimed at discovering the active ingredient in psychotherapy. Because all therapies were found to be effective, an important research question emerged: "What do all therapies have in common?" A number of common factors were found, of which the therapeutic relationship or therapeutic alliance is perhaps the most important (de Jonghe et al. 1992; Frank and Frank 1991; Rosenzweig 1936; Westerman et al. 1995). If there is a good alliance between patient and therapist, therapy is helpful. If there is not a good alliance, little is accomplished in therapy. Therefore, the therapist must make deliberate efforts to encourage a good relationship and avoid actions that are inimical to a good relationship. (See Chapter 6, "The Therapeutic Relationship," for further discussion.)

Alexander and French (1946) introduced the term *corrective emotional experience*. This comes about as the patient's transference may cause him or her to unconsciously perceive the therapist as having attributes associated with unpleasant interactions in the past. The therapist, however, does not respond as did the figure from the past, and in time, the old feelings become muted, and the patient no longer needs to replay new relationships according to the old emotional script. According to theory, this result is accomplished without explicit analysis. Corrective emotional experiences may occur at any point on the spectrum of psychopathology or the spectrum of psychotherapies. Gabbard (2010) summarizes current thinking: "Now most clinicians and researchers feel that insight through interpretation has historically been idealized and that change also occurs through the experience of a new kind of relationship in psychotherapy" (p. 94).

Education and instruction are potent agents for bringing about change in people's lives. Advice and instruction are most likely to be followed when given by a person the individual trusts and respects. The skillful therapist or teacher gives instruction that is needed at the time when it can be absorbed and used. The patient's mother may have said, "Clean your room." In contrast, the psychotherapist teaches, "It's not good for your self-esteem for you to be surrounded by evidence that you can't keep some order in your life." Sometimes, this approach is all that is required to bring about change.

In the 1960s, learning theory, which previously had been of more interest to science-minded psychologists than to clinical psychiatrists, was presented as the theoretical basis of behavior therapy (an approach that had been demonstrated to be effective for many disorders)—contrary to predictions based on theories underlying psychoanalytic therapy. Change, initiated by a therapy based on an educational approach, was found to occur even if neither patient nor therapist understood the historical origins of the problem. Education and instruction have been accepted throughout history as strategies for changing behavior and thought, although such changes cannot be guaranteed or predicted (it is remarkable how often, when a patient mentions a former therapist, the patient tells us what that therapist told him or her to do). Research on the process of learning, although focused on formal education, has led to observations that new information is linked to what is already known, that retrieving information repeatedly enhances subsequent recall, and that elaborating on the material contributes to learning (deWinstanley and Bjork 2002). Although the field of learning theory has contributed potentially useful ways of explaining the process of education and change, such as critical reflection (Mezirow 1998), these ideas have not percolated through psychotherapy education. The techniques of cognitive and behavior therapies are used somewhat informally in supportive psychotherapy, usually without the emphasis on homework. Faulty cognition and the persistence of automatic thoughts are recognized as processes that often contribute to symptom formation and to maladaptive behavior. In supportive psychotherapy, the therapist may address faulty cognition when the patient is able to accept the self-scrutiny entailed. Desensitization, a central theme of behavior therapy, may contribute to the beneficial effect of history-oriented psychotherapy in that it involves repeated safe exposure to once painful memories (Goldberg and Green 1986).

Patients at the most supportive end of the supportive-expressive continuum find that simply being able to talk to a person who is interested and accepting minimizes the loneliness in their lives; being able to talk about experiences and worries brings relief, even when the patients receive no reassuring or normalizing response. Identification with the therapist as a reasonable, stable individual may promote stability and better relationships with others. When associated with events that have been concealed, ventilation can be curative. Repeating the same story month after month may be comforting for the patient, even when he or she makes no progress. From the medical perspective, maintaining the status quo may be a reasonable and responsible objective. At the same time, however, therapists hope to find opportunities to help the patient improve his or her situation.

The concept of *change* appears throughout the literature on psychotherapy. At one end of the spectrum, change means lasting personality change. At the other end, desirable changes may involve specific behaviors, such as sitting in front of the television all day, skipping medications, spending money foolishly, remaining in a bad environment, or failing to control children. If simple advice is all that is needed to get the patient to change habitual behavior, it is not necessary to examine possible causes of the behavior. Often, however, there are obstacles to bringing about change that the patient does not verbalize. If the therapist is to give useful advice, he or she must be familiar with the psychological and emotional problems that may be operating.

Therapist 1: The last time you were here, we talked about the support group, and you said you were going to talk to the social worker about it. I wonder what happened that you didn't. *("What happened?" is not as attacking as "Why?")*
Patient 1: I don't know. I had trouble with my car. I had to go to the dentist.
Therapist 1: I know a lot of people have trouble doing too many things in one week. It's also an easy habit to get into and not a good one. *(Normalizing, exhorting, judgmental)*

Therapist 2: People who have not been able to do much for a long time—it can happen with illness—become fearful of doing new things. They think that they will do something wrong or won't know how to fit in. Does that make any sense? *(Teaching; confronting—i.e., bringing to the patient's attention feelings or thoughts that had been outside his or her awareness)*
Patient 2: I get very nervous when I meet new people.
Therapist 2: So we need to find a way to deal with the nervousness that will make it possible for you to have the interview with the social worker. Then you can determine whether the group might be of use to you. *(Scolding replaced by acceptance; moving toward constructive efforts)*

This dialogue illustrates how even in work with the most impaired individuals, the therapist must explore feelings and ideas of which the patient has not been aware. This exploration is an expressive element. If responsibility for the patient is to go beyond the simplest take-it-or-leave-it advice and beyond criticizing the patient for being noncompliant, the therapy must take into account psychodynamic considerations.

Films and plays of the 1950s often show a patient in psychotherapy or psychoanalysis discovering an early traumatic experience, after which recovery is immediate. However, in real life, once such discoveries are made, a patient typically must work hard to change his or her ways of thinking and responding. Although the importance of explaining origins is not as great as once thought, an explanation of origins still has its uses. For the patient to own a meaningful personal story is to give him or her a feeling of mastery, and the creation of the story is a shared task for patient and therapist. From the scientific point of view, the therapist can never be certain whether the patient's story agrees with what actually happened— or whether the apparent cause-and-effect connections are valid. As an example of the latter, people who have been beaten when they were children are more likely to be physically abusive adults than those who were never beaten—but this result is not inevitable. Therapists, as well as the general public, often blur the distinction between anecdote and group data. The methods of cognitive-behavioral therapy, many of which have been incorporated into supportive psychotherapy, may be the principal approach once the patient sees that the behavior that is causing the distress is the outcome of a plausible story.

Misch (2000) advises the supportive therapist to "be a good parent." Because patients operate ineffectively in one or more psychological domains, the therapist assumes a parental role in these domains. Parental behaviors include comforting, soothing, encouraging, nurturing, containment, limit setting, and confronting self-destructive behaviors, while all the time encouraging the patient's growth and self-sufficiency.

Conclusion

Supportive psychotherapy is conducted in conversational style, involving examination of the patient's current and past experiences, responses, and feelings. Although the initial focus is on self-esteem, ego function, and adaptive skills, the therapeutic alliance may be the most important element of the therapy. The therapist seeks to expand the patient's self-mastery by helping him or her to become aware of thoughts and feelings that had been outside awareness and to provide specific suggestions for more adaptive living.

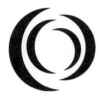

3

Assessment, Case Formulation, and Goal Setting

Assessment

The process of evaluation and case formulation is essential for all psychotherapeutic approaches. A central objective of the assessment process is to diagnose the patient's illness and describe the problems so that the patient can be treated appropriately. Another important objective of the evaluation process is to establish a therapeutic relationship, which can further the patient's interest in and commitment to psychotherapy. A thorough evaluation should help the clinician to select the appropriate treatment approach. The treatment plan should be individualized to meet the needs and goals of the patient.

The supportive-expressive continuum, introduced in Chapter 1, "The Concept of Supportive Psychotherapy," is a useful way of thinking about and conceptualizing the evaluation process. In this chapter, we combine the psychotherapy continuum (lower labels on Figure 3–1) with an impairment or psychopathology continuum (upper labels on Figure 3–1). Supportive psychotherapy is indicated for patients on the left side of the continuum (higher levels of psychopathology), whereas expressive psychotherapy is better suited for patients on the right side of the continuum (healthier patients).

When a therapist meets a patient for the first time, the therapist generally does not know the extent of the patient's impairment, psychopathology, or strengths. Therefore, the initial interview should begin with the therapist's attempting to understand why the patient has come for

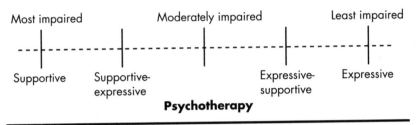

Figure 3–1. Impairment-psychotherapy continuum.

treatment. All patients should have a thorough evaluation of current problems and past history. However, the technical approach will vary from use of a more supportive approach for patients with higher levels of psychopathology to a more expressive approach for healthier patients. If the therapist, in the course of working with a patient, finds that the patient has more significant psychopathology, the therapist may have to quickly move into a more supportive mode. The degree of disturbance encountered during the initial interview will determine how the clinician proceeds in that interview.

The supportive-expressive psychotherapy continuum concept is the traditional way of thinking about dynamic psychotherapy. However, in our clinical and research work, we have found that supportive and expressive psychotherapies produce similar results in patients across the psychopathology continuum (see Chapter 9, "Evaluating Competence and Outcome Research"). The efficacy of supportive psychotherapy in higher-functioning patients is especially enhanced when expressive and cognitive-behavioral techniques are integrated into a supportive approach (Winston and Winston 2002). Therefore, supportive psychotherapy is indicated for a wide variety of disorders across the psychopathology continuum (see Chapter 5, "General Framework of Supportive Psychotherapy," for a full discussion of inclusion and exclusion criteria for supportive psychotherapy).

The evaluation should be comprehensive and, if possible, should be completed during an extended first session of at least 60 minutes. At the end of the evaluation, the therapist should understand the patient's problems, interpersonal relationships, everyday functioning, and psychological structure. The evaluation interview should not be a series of questions and answers but should be more of an exploration of the patient's life. The interview should be therapeutic, to help motivate the patient for treatment and promote the therapeutic alliance. In a supportive approach, a therapist may make an evaluation therapeutic by using appropriate interventions, such as empathic clarifications and confrontations.

The evaluation should begin with an exploration of the patient's presenting problems or areas of disturbance. Presenting problems may include symptoms, relationship and self difficulties, work or school issues, medical problems, and substance abuse issues. Generally, symptoms should be explored first so that the clinician is informed about the extent of the patient's psychopathology. Exploring symptoms first is also helpful to the patient because symptoms are what patients care about. Information about symptoms will enable the clinician to adjust the evaluation interview to the patient's level of psychopathology. When significant impairment exists, the interview should be more supportive, whereas with more cognitively intact patients, the interviewer can use an exploratory approach. With some patients, this distinction will be clear from the start, particularly if the patient has a loss of reality testing. With other patients, the extent of psychopathology may not be as readily discernible, so more time may be required to make this determination.

After the presenting problems have been clearly delineated, the therapist should explore the patient's history. This exploration can be done in many ways but should be systematic and should cover relationships with parents, other caretakers, siblings, grandparents, and other people in the patient's life and household; descriptions of these individuals should also be obtained. Important issues to inquire about include trauma, separation and loss, medical problems and psychiatric illness (in the patient and first-degree relatives), geographic moves, family belief systems, school history, sexual development and experiences, identity issues, and financial matters. Past psychiatric treatment, including psychotherapy and pharmacotherapy, should be explored, as should the patient's response to the therapist, because this knowledge can alert the therapist to potential problems in the therapeutic alliance.

As soon as the therapist determines that the patient should be treated with supportive or supportive-expressive psychotherapy, the evaluation interview should promote the objectives of supportive psychotherapy. These objectives are to ameliorate symptoms and to maintain, restore, or improve self-esteem, adaptive skills, and ego or psychological functions (Pinsker et al. 1991).

A useful method of conceptualizing dynamic psychotherapy, which encompasses both supportive and expressive approaches, involves the triangles of conflict and person. The focus of the triangle of conflict (Freud 1926/1959; Malan 1979) (Figure 3–2) is on wishes, needs, and feelings that are warded off by defenses and anxiety. In this model, a therapist who is pursuing a patient's feeling is at the wish/need/feeling point of the triangle. As is often the case, the patient may respond defensively to the exploration of feeling.

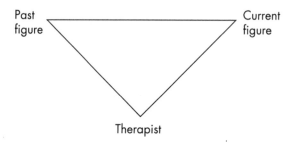

Figure 3–2. Triangle of person.

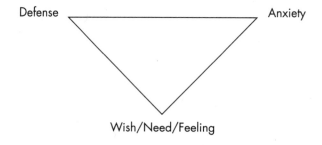

Figure 3–3. Triangle of conflict.

Defense is the second point of the triangle. The patient also may respond with anxiety because of fear of the conflicted feeling. Anxiety is the third point of this triangle. In the triangle of person (Malan 1979; Menninger 1958) (Figure 3–3), the three points all relate to people: individuals in the patient's current life and past life and the therapist or transference figure.

In expressive or exploratory psychotherapy, the therapist tends to work on conflict situations using the triangles to explore wishes, needs, and feelings that the patient may have in relation to an important person in his or her life. When defenses interfere with exploration, the therapist addresses them. Additionally, present and past issues are addressed, and the transference relationship and its exploration are emphasized.

In supportive psychotherapy, the triangles of conflict and person are used differently. In the triangle of conflict, feelings generally are not pursued, anxiety is diminished, and defenses are strengthened. In the triangle of person, the real relationship with the therapist is emphasized, and the therapist works primarily on present persons and current issues in the patient's life.

The following vignette, presented as an enactment on the accompanying DVD, illustrates use of supportive therapy in an initial evaluation (see Vignette 1 on the DVD).

▶ Vignette 1: Assessment

Mary, a 42-year-old woman, was referred by her primary care physician because of depression, beginning at age 24, and a number of other problems. She recently went through a divorce and is having a great deal of difficulty finding a job. She has a history of multiple episodes of depression and was hospitalized once for suicidal depression.

Therapist: As you know, Dr. Perry sent you to see me for an evaluation. Can you tell me what the problem is?

Mary: I just don't feel right. I don't know. ... I can't seem to get anything done. *(Responds in a vague manner that could be defensive or a sign of disorganization)*

Therapist: So you don't feel right and you haven't been able to get anything done and you're at a loss. *(Responds with a supportive clarification that helps Mary to focus on the question at hand)*

Mary: Yeah, I just sit around. ... I can't get started. ... Everything is just a mess. I feel so bad. *[becomes tearful]*

The therapist recognizes that the patient may be depressed and asks a series of questions to determine whether the patient is depressed and the extent of the depression.

- Have you been feeling down? Have you been crying or feeling tearful?
- What is your energy level like? Have you been tired a lot?
- Are you anxious, fearful, jumpy?
- What about your sleep patterns? Are you having problems falling asleep or are you sleeping too much?
- How is your appetite? Are you losing or gaining weight?
- Are you maintaining your social relationships? Do you find pleasure in your life? Do you go out?
- What is your attitude about the future? Do you feel hopeful?
- Have you wished you were dead or wished you could go to sleep and not wake up? Have you had any thoughts of killing yourself? Have you been thinking about how you might do this? Have you had these thoughts and had some intention of acting on them (Posner et al. 2009)?
- Are you able to have sexual relations? Is sex pleasurable?

▶ Vignette 1: Assessment *(continued)*

Mary responds that for the past 2 months, she has been consistently downhearted, tearful, fatigued, and pessimistic about the future and has had difficulty concentrating. She has trouble falling asleep, consistently awakens during early morning hours, and is unable to get back to sleep. Her appetite is poor, and she has lost approximately 10 pounds in the past 2 weeks. She is preoccupied with death and has thoughts of killing herself but no defined plan. She rarely goes out, nothing gives her pleasure or satisfaction, and she has no sexual desire or interest. She has never had a manic or hypomanic episode. In the past, she was treated with antidepressants, and during her last episode, she was treated with paroxetine. Mary stopped taking her medication 6 months ago.

The therapist recognizes that the patient is in the midst of a major depressive episode and has some cognitive difficulties. This level of psychopathology places Mary on the left side of the continuum, which indicates that the therapist should continue the evaluation in a supportive mode.

> Therapist: So it sounds to me as if you've been feeling depressed. From what you've told me, it seems you're depressed now and have been depressed several times in the past. These things you're describing—tearfulness, fatigue, difficulty concentrating, trouble sleeping, feeling bad, having a hard time getting started—all these things are symptoms of depression. *(Naming the problem makes it understandable and reassures patient that each symptom is not a separate condition.)*

The therapist has begun to educate the patient about her depression. Education is important in all forms of psychotherapy, but especially in supportive treatment. Education provides the patient with knowledge about his or her difficulties and also demonstrates the therapist's interest and understanding, thereby promoting the therapeutic alliance. Next, the therapist explores how the current episode of depression began.

> Mary: I just feel so hopeless and horrible. I feel like nothing's ever going to get better.... It's just that there are so many things...so many things that are bothering me.
> Therapist: We should try to look at this episode of depression. How long ago did it start? *(Proposed agenda)*
> Mary: Ah.... It got really bad 2 months ago...but I have to tell you I haven't been feeling well probably for the past year. I don't feel myself.
> Therapist: Did anything in particular happen? *(Continues to focus)*

▶ **Vignette 1: Assessment** *(continued)*

Mary: My husband…Edward, who I've been married to for 14 years… I just found out that he had an affair with this woman that he works with…and he had the affair and left me. *[tearful]* That's all I can say. **(Begins to reveal important material that may have contributed to onset of her depression)**

Therapist: I can see that this is really hard for you. **(Empathic support)**

Mary: It's worse…I don't know what I did wrong…I feel so stupid… I feel I can't do anything…I can't go to work…I can't face the people. The people at work will think that I'm pathetic, and I'm too ashamed to tell anyone. I don't like to talk about it. **(Indicates that her husband's infidelity and leaving her led to a series of automatic thoughts)**

Therapist: So have you been able to continue at your job? **(Early focus on adaptive activity)**

Mary: Well, it's been a struggle. It has been really hard.

Therapist: What do you think your coworkers might be thinking about you? **(Begins to explore Mary's automatic thoughts)**

Mary: They think I'm pathetic.… I used to call my husband all the time from work.… I felt so lonely and I felt so scared that I couldn't do things right…and he would get so angry at me and he would say, "Why are you calling me? Why are you bothering me? Can't you do anything for yourself?"

Therapist: You've been feeling incompetent?

Mary: I feel so incompetent and…

Therapist: Can you give me a specific example of this? **(Asks for a specific example. Remaining at an abstract or general level promotes vagueness and loss of focus.)**

Mary: Oh, God…I mean…I was feeling incompetent. I remember this one time…when I was at work…and I fell and hit my head, and my head was bleeding and I needed stitches, and I called my husband to come help me and bring me to the doctor to get stitches, and he got angry at me and told me that he was busy and not to bother him…and that I can't do anything right. I just felt so useless after that. **(Provides a clear interpersonal example)**

Therapist: So you reached out to your husband for help and not only did he not help you but he also put you down for it. This contributed to making you feel incompetent? **(Summarizes patient's story)**

Mary: Well, yeah.… I can't do anything right. I can't do anything right…yeah.

Therapist: I think that most people in that situation would ask for help and reach out to somebody. So I think that maybe you are making an erroneous judgment about yourself. **(Normalizing and then clarifying Mary's automatic thinking)**

Mary: You think so?

▶ **Vignette 1: Assessment** *(continued)*

Therapist: Perhaps this is a pattern with you? *(Asks if this might be her habitual manner of behaving)*
Mary: Maybe…I don't know?

The therapist has elicited a concrete example of an interaction with the patient's husband, an interaction that led the patient to think of herself as incompetent and helpless. This way of thinking is an example of automatic thoughts, which are quite common in depression. Mary's thought processes would constitute an important area on which to concentrate in supportive therapy for this type of disorder. In this instance, the therapist has attempted to point out that Mary's negative thinking was faulty, but the therapist has done so in a supportive manner by asking if Mary agreed. In subsequent sessions, the therapist should help the patient to test her automatic thoughts herself.

The therapist then goes on to explore the patient's relationship with Edward, the history of their marriage, and Mary's past history.

The patient is in the throes of a major depressive disorder and has had four previous major depressive episodes, as well as a milder, chronic depression for most of her life. Serious difficulties in the interpersonal sphere, as well as personality problems, limit her ability to function. The therapist, a psychiatrist, concluded that Mary would benefit from medication and a supportive psychotherapy approach employing cognitive-behavioral techniques. The therapist explained how both approaches—medication and psychotherapy—would be helpful in treating Mary's depression, anxiety, and problems in day-to-day functioning. The patient agreed with these immediate treatment goals and stated that she thought the medication and psychotherapy were worth a try. An explanation was given about when the medication would begin to work and would have maximum effect. In addition, possible side effects of the medication were discussed.

Diagnostic Evaluation

- Axis I: Major depressive disorder, recurrent
- Axis II: Dependent personality disorder
- Axis III: None
- Axis IV: Loss of husband
- Axis V: Global Assessment of Functioning=55

Case Formulation

For each patient, the treatment approach should be based on the central issues emerging from the assessment and case formulation. Case formulation depends on an accurate and thorough assessment of the patient. The *case formulation* is an explanation of the patient's symptoms and psychosocial functioning. The therapist's formulation governs what interventions will be used as well as which issues in the patient-therapist dialogue will be selected for attention. Having a sense of the underlying issues at the start enhances the therapist's ability to respond empathically. At the same time, empathy for the patient helps the therapist to guide and plan therapy effectively. The initial formulation is tentative and must be modified as more is learned about the patient during the course of psychotherapy.

Although the DSM diagnosis (American Psychiatric Association 2000) is an important element of the formulation, it is by no means the whole story. It does not illuminate an individual's adaptive or maladaptive characteristics, such as disappointments, the capacity for relationships, and how the individual thinks about and interprets life's events. Nor does the diagnosis explain the unique life history of an individual. The DSM diagnosis alone does not explain the patient or the problem.

In the following subsections, we discuss the following case formulation approaches: structural, genetic, dynamic, and cognitive-behavioral (Table 3–1). Supportive psychotherapy uses elements of all these approaches but differs in how these elements are used. For example, a patient's conflict may be clearly understood and formulated by the therapist but never or only partially explored in psychotherapy. Although these approaches have always been described separately, a great deal of overlap exists, so some repetition occurs in the descriptions.

Structural Approach

A structural case formulation (Table 3–2) attempts to capture the relatively fixed characteristics of an individual's personality, which is understood within a functional context (in contrast with genetic and dynamic approaches, which are more content based). Assessment of an individual's strengths and weaknesses and overall level of psychopathology helps determine the clinician's choice of technical approaches. A thorough structural assessment enables the clinician to determine with some degree of accuracy where to place the patient on the psychopathological–psychological structure continuum (see Figure 3–1).

Structural functions have been grouped together using Freud's (1923/ 1961) structural approach of id, ego, and superego. These agencies refer to

Table 3–1. Types and foci of case formulations

Type	Focus
Structural	Concentrates on fixed aspects of an individual's personality within a functional context; assesses strengths and weaknesses and overall level of psychopathology
Genetic	Explores early development and life events that may explain the patient's current situation
Dynamic	Highlights the content of an individual's current conflicts and relates it to a primary lifelong or core conflict; examines mental and/or emotional tensions that may be conscious or unconscious
Cognitive-behavioral	Attends to the individual's automatic thoughts (based on the person's core beliefs or negative schemas) and how they can be addressed to change thoughts, behaviors, and moods

the inner life of the patient. The following description of psychological or ego functions is based on the work of Beres (1956) and Bellak (1958). These categories are not mutually exclusive; there is a great deal of overlap.

Relation to Reality

Beres (1956) and Bellak (1958) described reality testing and sense of reality as major components of relation to reality. The term *reality testing* describes an individual's ability to assess reality. Reality testing is impaired in the presence of faulty judgment and is grossly disturbed in the presence of hallucinations or delusions. Sense of reality relates to a person's ability to distinguish self from other; presence of this ability indicates a stable and cohesive body image. Examples of disturbances in this function are depersonalization, derealization, and identity problems.

Disturbances in relation to reality indicate significant structural problems that place the patient on the left side of the psychopathological–psychological structure continuum, and such disturbances should point the clinician in the direction of a more supportive approach. Impaired relation to reality is a key indicator of structural deficits and should always be thoroughly explored.

Object Relations

The term *object relations* refers to a person's capacity to relate in a meaningful way to significant individuals in his or her life. The function includes the ability to form intimate relationships, tolerate separation and loss, and maintain independence and autonomy. It also involves the sense

Table 3–2. Components of the structural approach (ego and superego)

Ego functions	Ego functions *(continued)*
Relation to reality	Autonomous functions (perception, intention, intelligence, language, and motor development)
Object relations	
Affects	Synthetic function (ability to form a cohesive whole or gestalt)
Impulse control	
Defenses	**Superego functions**
Thought processes	Conscience, morals, and ideals

of self and the ability to form a cohesive and stable self-image without diminishing or overidealizing self or other.

A patient's relationships with others form the foundation of the psychological functions constituting the structural approach. In all forms of psychotherapy, evaluation of object relations is central in determining a patient's placement on the psychopathological–psychological structure continuum. Patients who are withdrawn and not interested in others or who have narcissistic, highly dependent, or chaotic relationships generally require a more supportive approach and therefore are on the left side of the continuum. Individuals who have had at least one meaningful give-and-take relationship tend to be on the right side of the continuum.

Affects, Impulse Control, and Defenses

Affects are complex psychophysiological states composed of subjective feelings and physiological accompaniments such as crying, blushing, sweating, posture, facial expression, and tone of voice. The range of affects includes excitement, joy, surprise, fear, anger, rage, irritation, anguish, shame, humiliation, sadness, and depression. The individual's ability to experience a wide range of affects at some depth and to differentiate between affects (as opposed to lumping them into a single feeling such as primitive rage) need to be assessed. Does the individual experience a wide variety and range of affects, and is the individual able to tolerate love, anger, joy, sadness, and humiliation? What are the predominant affects (Friedman and Lister 1987), and how regularly are they invoked?

The capacity to control impulses and to modulate affect in an adaptive manner indicates a well-functioning defensive structure. When impulse control is faulty, the individual may engage in socially unacceptable behavior, such as physically or verbally lashing out at others or making inappropriate demands. The ability to delay gratification and to tolerate frustration is another important aspect of impulse control.

Defenses mediate between a person's wishes, needs, and feelings and both internal prohibitions and the external world. Individuals tend to use the same kinds of behavior as patterned responses in reaction to perceived danger, difficult situations, or painful affects. Defenses are conceptualized as having both a developmental and a hierarchical organization. Three levels of defenses have been described: immature, intermediate, and mature. Some immature defenses are projection, hypochondriasis, acting out, sarcasm, and avoidance. Intermediate defenses include forgetting, intellectualization, displacement, and rationalization. Among the mature defenses are altruism, anticipation, suppression, sublimation, and humor (Vaillant 1977, 1986). Primitive defenses, poor impulse control, severe affective instability, and shallow affect are indicators of structural deficits that place an individual on the left side of the continuum and suggest the need for a more supportive approach.

Thought Processes

The ability to think clearly, logically, and abstractly should be assessed. High levels of primary process or primitive thinking are a good indicator of severe psychopathology. Significant limitations in the ability to think logically suggest the need for a more supportive approach as opposed to an exploratory one. Dysfunctional and automatic thoughts should be identified so that cognitive-behavioral approaches can be applied.

Autonomous Functions

Autonomous functions—perception, intention, intelligence, language, and motor development—are believed to develop in a relatively conflict-free manner (Hartmann 1939/1958). Although these functions generally are not impaired in patients on the right side of the psychopathological–psychological structure continuum, the functions can be affected in patients with significant psychopathology.

Synthetic Function

Synthetic function (Nunberg 1931) is the individual's ability to organize himself or herself and the world in a productive manner. It is the psychological ability to form a cohesive whole, or gestalt, by putting together the other functions and organizing them, so that the person can function in a harmonious and integrated way. For example, a young man meets several men and women for the first time at a dinner party. He engages each individual in a friendly and open manner with an appropriate affect. He is thoughtful, coherent, and humorous. In this example, the young man synthesizes the ego functions of object relations (friendly and open), appropriate affect, thoughtfulness and coherence, and a high level defense or coping style of humor.

Conscience, Morals, and Ideals

Conscience, morals, and ideals derive from internalization of aspects of parental figures and social mores. Freud (1926/1959) conceptualized these elements as aspects of the superego. Severe impairments in these functions can interfere with the patient-therapist relationship. For instance, if a patient is not truthful with the therapist, achieving success in psychotherapy may be difficult.

Case Illustration: Structural Case Formulation

The following case provides the basis for a structural case formulation.

> Bert, a 24-year-old man with panic disorder, has developed the belief that his coworkers are saying derogatory things about him and want to hurt him physically. His relationships are characterized by an absence of concern for self or others, and this lack of concern often puts him at risk. He uses women to satisfy his sexual needs, abruptly leaving them and giving untruthful excuses. At times he becomes enraged with and is physically abusive toward them. His aggressive and violent behavior evokes fears of retaliation. He both uses and sells drugs. The patient has a history of beginning schools and jobs, quitting them when he encounters difficulties, and blaming others for his failures.

Bert has impaired reality testing, consisting of ideas about others talking and plotting against him. His adaptive skills are poor, as demonstrated by his inability to work or to complete school. Relationships are conducted on a need-satisfying basis, without concern for others. Bert is often sadistic but then becomes self-defeating and self-punishing. He exhibits impaired frustration tolerance and poorly controlled impulses, and his displays of rage may indicate a limited repertoire of affective responses. He uses immature defenses, such as projection, acting out, and denial.

Genetic Approach

The genetic area of case formulation involves exploration of early development and life events that may help to explain an individual's current situation. Genetics are the genesis of the dynamics. Life presents many challenges, conflicts, and crises. These can be traumatic, depending on their severity, the developmental stage of the child, and the quality of his or her support system. Events or conditions that need to be considered as important in a child's development include the loss of a significant person, separation, abuse, the birth of a sibling, birth defects and developmental deficits, learning problems, illness, surgery, and substance abuse. A single event can have a traumatic effect on an individual, although often it is the day-to-day negative experiences that lead to significant conflict, psychopathology, and characterological problems. Examples of day-to-day events are constant criticism, devaluing, abusive behavior, parental conflict, and significant psychiatric problems. The genetic approach follows the development of the child from birth to late adolescence or early adulthood.

An example of a persistent difficulty or traumatic situation is the experience of a young boy growing up with a violent alcoholic father who is demeaning and at times physically abusive. Persistent trauma such as that caused by unresponsiveness of a parent may be more subtle and difficult to evaluate. For instance, a narcissistic mother may use her daughter for her own self-enhancement. She may ignore her child's real qualities, demanding behavior the child is unable to deliver or can deliver only at considerable cost to herself.

Dynamic Approach

The dynamic approach is useful with mental and/or emotional tensions that may be conscious or unconscious. The therapist using this approach focuses on conflicting wishes, needs, or feelings, and their meanings. In a conflict situation, an individual wards off or defends against wishes, needs, or feelings. The dynamic approach highlights the content of an individual's current conflicts and relates it to a primary lifelong or core conflict (Perry et al. 1987).

In contrast to structural case formulation, which is based on an individual's relatively fixed characteristics and functioning, dynamic case formulation is concerned with meaning and content. The dynamic approach focuses on current conflicts, whereas the genetic approach focuses on a person's developmental history, including childhood and adolescent traumas and conflicts and their possible meanings. Childhood conflicts tend to be revived and relived in adult life.

A useful approach to understanding the dynamics of an individual, particularly the core conflict, involves mapping the central relationship patterns. An understanding of these patterns requires exploration of three aspects of interpersonal interactions: 1) what the person wants from others, 2) how others react to the person, and 3) how the person responds to others' reactions. These categories form the basis of the core conflictual relationship theme (CCRT) method, an approach that relies on "narratives, called relationship episodes, that patients typically tell and sometimes even enact during their psychotherapy session" (Luborsky and

Crits-Christoph 1990, p. 15). The CCRT is composed of the patient's wishes or needs of others and how others respond (their actual responses as well as their responses from the patient's perspective). Understanding and using the CCRT method provides the clinician with a central organizing focus. The CCRT method can be used differentially with patients according to their position on the continuum.

Case Illustration: Dynamic Case Formulation

The following case illustrates a dynamic conflict as well as its genetic or historical basis.

> Tim is a passive 48-year-old man whose father has become increasingly debilitated and demanding, a state made worse by early signs of dementia. His father often telephones with complaints and demands, even though Tim has been consistently helpful. After these calls, Tim finds himself wishing that his father appreciated him. He becomes anxiety ridden and often is angry with his wife and friends, later feeling guilty about his behavior. At work, he has become increasingly anxious and perfectionistic, and he worries that his boss dislikes him and will criticize him.
>
> The dynamic explanation is that Tim has ambivalent feelings toward his father, consisting of anger and possibly a wish for his father to die, combined with positive feelings based on earlier experiences. He becomes anxious and defends against these feelings or wishes by displacing the anger he feels toward his father onto his wife and friends. The anxiety serves as a signal of unacceptable feelings. His boss is viewed as an authority figure and has become linked with his father, who is both loved and hated. In general, Tim is passive and avoids confrontation. He fears making a mistake and being humiliated. According to the CCRT method, Tim's wish to be appreciated by his father can be identified. The response of the other, his father, is lack of appreciation combined with hostility, and the response of the self is displacement of anger onto Tim's wife and friends and feeling unappreciated. The genetic basis of Tim's current conflict is related to his experiencing his father as being both highly critical, and concerned and loving to him when he was a youngster. This early experience has resulted in mixed feelings toward his father, consisting of love and rage with accompanying anxiety, guilt, and lack of assertiveness.

Cognitive-Behavioral Approach

Although case formulation has not been widely used in cognitive-behavioral therapy, models have been developed that are helpful in assessing an individual's problems in cognition (Persons 1989, 1993). Cognitive-behavioral therapy is initially directed at automatic thoughts, which are based on core beliefs or negative schemas. Overt and underlying beliefs are closely linked and are expressed as thoughts, behaviors, and moods. Core beliefs are addressed later in the course of therapy. The cognitive-behavioral case formulation model, as adapted from Tompkins (1996), has the following components:

1. Problem list (including automatic thoughts)
2. Core beliefs
3. Origins
4. Precipitants and activating situations
5. Predicted obstacles to treatment
6. Treatment plan

The description of Tim (see "Case Illustration: Dynamic Case Formulation" in the previous section) will be used to illustrate these six components of cognitive-behavioral case formulations.

The *problem list* is a complete list of the patient's difficulties and presenting complaints. It includes the dysfunctional thinking responsible for the maladaptive behavior and disturbed mood. Tim's mood problems are anxiety, anger, and feelings of guilt. His problematic behavior is his inappropriate rage at his wife and friends. His automatic thoughts ("I am flawed" and "I will make mistakes and be humiliated") lead to passivity and lack of assertiveness.

Core beliefs are hypotheses about the patient's self-schemas and views of others and the world. Tim's core belief is a pervasive sense that he cannot do anything right. This belief makes him especially vulnerable to the opinions of others. The *origins* of core beliefs are early experiences, generally involving parents or parental figures. Tim's core beliefs appear to have derived from his relationship with his overly critical father.

Core beliefs are generally *activated by situations or events* that are stressful or problematic for the patient. The deteriorating health of his father precipitated Tim's current difficulty and brought him into treatment.

Obstacles to treatment should be anticipated if possible. Obstacles in Tim's case might be reflected in the patient-therapist relationship. Fear of criticism can emerge in relation to the therapist and lead to increased patient passivity in the treatment situation. Tim may be reluctant to complete homework assignments because he fears that the therapist will be critical.

A well-conceived and comprehensive *treatment plan* should emerge from the case formulation. This plan should include goals and the types of interventions to be used. For Tim, the goals should include decreasing his anxiety, reducing or eliminating his anger toward his wife and friends, and decreasing his difficulties at work. The interventions should consist of cognitive restruturing of Tim's thinking about his father and relaxation therapy to reduce anxiety.

The Four Approaches Compared and Applied

A number of similarities exist among the structural, genetic, dynamic, and cognitive-behavioral approaches as used in dynamic (supportive and expressive) and cognitive-behavioral therapies. The concept of core beliefs and their origins is similar to the idea of the genetic case formulation, which provides the origins of structural and dynamic factors. The notion of activating events in cognitive-behavioral therapy is analogous to the precipitation of genetic and dynamic conflicts. Obstacles to treatment often relate to the therapeutic relationship, and thus the concept of obstacles is similar in genetic and dynamic approaches. Cognitive-behavioral therapy adds a different dimension to case formulation and the treatment approach, particularly when thinking problems are present. Dynamic and genetic approaches do not involve a major focus on thinking, but the structural approach does include evaluation of an individual's thought processes.

Following are case formulations and diagnostic assessments of Mary, the patient evaluated in "Vignette 1: Assessment" in the "Assessment" section earlier in this chapter.

Structural Approach

Mary is an intelligent woman with limited insight and judgment. Although her reality testing is intact, her adaptive skills are impaired. She has difficulty functioning, caring for herself, and working. Her object relations are on a need-satisfying level. Mary has low self-esteem, a result of early experiences with her mother and sisters and more recent experiences with her husband. Her depression has intensified her feelings of inadequacy. The defenses Mary uses are at the immature level and consist of avoidance, denial, and projection. Predominant affects are sadness and anger. Mary has many negative thoughts about herself and is somewhat impulsive.

Genetic Approach

Mary is the youngest of three girls born to older parents. Her parents did not expect a third child, and her mother considered aborting the pregnancy. Mary grew up with a sense of not being wanted by her mother. Mary felt she was the least favored child compared with her sisters, who were admired by their mother for their intelligence and beauty. Her mother's attitude toward Mary interfered with her development of a positive self-image, resulting in faltering self-esteem. When Mary was 14 years old, her father—with whom she had a predominantly positive relationship—suddenly died. At that time, her mother became less available and was more critical of Mary. The death of her father, who had been a source of comfort during her adolescence, may have added to her impaired self-esteem and her neediness.

Dynamic Approach

Mary is a needy, dependent woman who wishes to be cared for. The patient's core conflict revolves around her wish to be wanted and cared for by others (mother and husband). When the response of others is to abandon her (father's death), criticize her, or favor others (sisters and husband's lover), she becomes depressed and withdrawn, with diminished self-esteem. Her wish to be cared for is an expression of her need to feel she has a right to exist.

Cognitive-Behavioral Approach

Mary's problems include depression, interpersonal difficulties with her husband and coworkers, and an inability to maintain day-to-day functioning. Her automatic thoughts—"I can't do anything right" and "I need someone to care for me"—are based on Mary's core beliefs that she is worthless, a failure, and in need of constant support, without which she cannot function. The origins of her core beliefs are her mother's and sisters' view that she was weak, sickly, and not as capable as her sisters.

Precipitants of and activating situations for Mary's difficulties are the loss of her husband and the discontinuation of her medication for previous depression. The obstacles to treatment are Mary's severe neediness and her fear that the therapist will view her as inadequate.

Goal Setting

For patients requiring supportive psychotherapy, organizing goals should be as follows:

1. Amelioration of symptoms
2. Improvement of adaptation
3. Enhancement of self-esteem
4. Improvement of overall functioning

Setting goals in psychotherapy is important in guiding the treatment, because both therapist and patient must agree on the objectives of treatment. The goals set within the first few sessions should be viewed as preliminary and open to change. Both immediate objectives for each session and ultimate goals (Parloff 1967) for treatment should be considered. For example, an immediate in-session objective for Mary might be to develop a mutually agreed-on plan for helping her return to work within a week. An ultimate goal for her would be to promote job stability and improve relationships with coworkers.

Clearly outlined goals help motivate patients and promote the therapeutic alliance as patient and therapist work toward a common end. The goals of treatment should be derived from the patient's problem areas so that motivation to change will be enhanced and will promote therapeutic clarity. These goals are different from the goals of expressive psychotherapy, which are symptom and personality change through analysis of the patient-therapist relationship and through development of insight into previously unrecognized feelings, thoughts, needs, and conflicts.

An assumption in the past was that long-term changes in conflicts and personality cannot occur in supportive psychotherapy. However, results of studies by Rosenthal et al. (1999) and Winston et al. (2001) suggested that supportive psychotherapy can produce personality changes in patients on the healthier side of the impairment–psychotherapy continuum.

The goals of therapy should generally be the patient's. In the event of disagreement on goals, the therapist enters into an exploration of the problem. In the case of Mary, one of the mutually agreed-on goals was to resolve her depression and to prevent future episodes of depression. However, during Mary's previous episodes of depression, she stopped taking her medication when she was no longer depressed. Therefore, an important goal for Mary is to continue taking her medication to help prevent future depressive episodes. After the therapist explored the reasons Mary stopped taking her medication and educated her about the risks of discontinuing, she agreed with this treatment goal.

Setting realistic goals is important, especially with patients who have severe psychopathology. Some patients may have grandiose fantasies or magical wishes that need to be modified. Mary had the unrealistic expectation that her husband would return to her, which she thought would solve her problems.

Treatment goals should never be regarded as fixed and unchangeable. For example, once Mary's depression is resolved, she may want help with expanding her social network and improving her interpersonal relationships.

Conclusion

Assessment of the patient's problems, symptoms, and character structure is critical for arriving at a complete diagnosis, case formulation, and treatment plan. Case formulation should be comprehensive—encompassing structural, genetic, dynamic, and cognitive-behavioral approaches. We have illustrated this process by presenting a case example from an initial assessment and case formulation of a patient, as well as describing the setting of treatment goals for this patient.

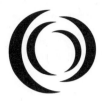

4

Techniques

In Chapter 2, "Principles and Mode of Action," we described the following as principles of supportive psychotherapy: 1) the interaction between patient and therapist is conversational; and 2) the transferential aspects of the relationship are subordinate to the reality aspects of the relationship. Rosenthal (2009) characterized these principles as "contextual techniques" because they underlie all supportive psychotherapy. In this chapter, we describe specific techniques (Table 4–1) that are *interventions* (a term often used to describe the actions of a therapist). These techniques are employed to maintain the therapeutic alliance—without which nothing can be accomplished—and to achieve the objectives of supportive psychotherapy (described in Chapter 1, "The Concept of Supportive Psychotherapy"): maintaining or improving self-esteem, ego function, and adaptive skills.

Alliance Building

Because the therapeutic alliance has been demonstrated to be one of most critical predictors, if not the most critical predictor, of the outcome of any form of psychotherapy (Horvath and Symmonds 1991; Westerman et al. 1995), the therapist using supportive psychotherapy should purposefully set out to build and maintain this alliance. To support the alliance, the therapist expresses interest, empathy, and understanding. The therapist makes comments to sustain conversation and, thus, the connection between patient and therapist. When the therapist suspects that the pa-

---

Table 4–1. Supportive psychotherapy techniques

Alliance building	**Reducing and preventing anxiety**
Expressions of interest	Conversational style
Expressions of empathy	Sharing the agenda
Expressions of understanding	Verbal "padding"
Sustaining comments	Naming the problem
Conversational style	Normalizing
Repair of misalliance	Reframing
Esteem building	Rationalizing
Praise	**Awareness expanding**
Reassurance	Clarification
Normalizing	Confrontation
Universalizing	Interpretation
Encouragement	
Exhortation	
Skills building—adaptive behavior	
Advice	
Teaching	
Modeling adaptive behavior	
Anticipatory guidance	

---

tient's positive feelings about him or her are unrealistic, possibly a product of transference, the matter is not discussed. Threats to the alliance are always a concern, whether the cause is life circumstances, misinformation, the therapist's actual behavior, or transference. Attention to misalliance and to repair of ruptures in the relationship is important and is discussed more fully in Chapter 6, "The Therapeutic Relationship."

The beginning therapist may not know what to talk about with a new patient. A good place to start is with what the patient wants to talk about, but then the therapist must decide whether to dwell on that topic or move to others that experience has indicated are often fruitful or important. For example, when the patient has recently been hospitalized, medications are a priority topic. The first questions are whether the patient is taking medications regularly and whether he or she is experiencing any unwanted or uncomfortable effects. When patients do not take medication as prescribed, physicians often accuse the patients of being noncompliant. Focusing on untoward effects helps to transform the matter from adversarial to collaborative. Later, the therapist can broach psychological issues that might affect willingness to take medication. Possible issues include not wanting to feel overpowered by medication and not wanting to accept the existence of illness.

The therapist should discuss details of daily life with the nonfunctioning individual and should seek opportunities to discuss the patient's adaptive skills. The therapist should make an effort to know how the patient understands his or her condition and what feelings are related to it. A person who has a chronic disabling condition ought to have the opportunity to talk about it. The patient may have fears about the future that are not expressed. Depression accompanies many conditions. Depression may be a patient's response to discovering that he or she faces a life of disability or a response to looking back over lost years and family tension.

The therapist should know about the people in the patient's life. Higher-functioning patients are likely to have important relationships, to think about their interactions, and to bring them up for discussion. Lower-functioning patients (and some elderly patients) may lead lives almost devoid of relationships and may talk at length about their symptoms or abstractly about their mental problems. The therapist should make an effort to know about family, friends, acquaintances, coworkers, and in the case of an isolated patient, persons with whom the patient has even brief contacts, such as caseworkers, probation officers, receptionists, guards, and food servers.

Therapist 1: Did you have contact with anyone in the last few days?
Patient 1: My sister-in-law called.
Therapist 1: Tell me about her.
Patient 1: She's gross.
Therapist 1: Can you describe her? *(A broader and less demanding question than "Why don't you like her?")*

Therapist 2: Who are the people in your life now?
Patient 2: No one. The only people I know use drugs.
Therapist 2: Is there someone you talk to most days?

Therapist 3: You say your son will come if you call him. Does that mean he doesn't come if you don't call?
Patient 3: He'll drop what he's doing if we need him, but...to come on a Sunday afternoon? Forget it.

Therapist 4: Tell me about the people who live in the residence.

Therapist 5: Girlfriend? Is this someone you've known for some time?

Some well-spoken or well-educated patients ruminate endlessly and unproductively about their introspections and their speculations about the childhood origins of their trouble, without ever saying a word about current activity or people.

Esteem Building

The supportive techniques of praise, reassurance, and encouragement are directed primarily to self-esteem concerns. By his or her attitude, the therapist conveys his or her acceptance, respect, and interest.

Praise

A good supportive technique is to express praise when the patient has accomplished something. Praise can be interspersed throughout a conversation, sprinkled in like salt from a saltshaker. Praise may reinforce the patient's accomplishments or improvement in adaptive efforts, provided that the patient is likely to agree that the praise is deserved.

> Therapist 1: Telling your mother that you knew you had been nasty was a good step. Do you agree?
> Therapist 2: You're able to make this very clear.
> Therapist 3: It's good that you can be so considerate of other people. *(Note, however, that in some contexts, being too considerate may be seen as a symptom, and a statement that the patient is considerate might be presented as a confrontation.)*

False praise or praise that is meaningless to the patient is worse than saying nothing. Falsity and deception are incompatible with any good relationship.

> Patient: I was always afraid of my mother.
> Therapist: What were you afraid of?
> Patient: She came in this morning and said, "Why are you still in bed?" She doesn't respect me. They argue a lot. I was 15 before I realized that she was crazy.
> Therapist 1: You explained that well. *(A supportive comment, but in this instance false praise. Patient has mixed past and present, his mother's attitude toward him, and her relationship with her husband. Thought-disordered responses can be "decoded," but patient cannot be said to have explained the situation well.)*
> Therapist 2: It's hard for you to describe these things. You're making a big effort. *(Accurate and useful)*

When the therapist expresses praise for something that the patient cannot feel good about, his or her words will be ineffective and may even have a negative impact.

> Patient: I really have been feeling bad. I don't do anything. I manage to eat, but most of the time I'm a blob.
> Therapist 1: Did you do anything last week besides sit around at home? *(Not content with global self-description, seeks specifics)*

Patient: Well, I went to a movie…
Therapist 1: That's great!!!
Patient: Yeah.
(Therapist didn't appreciate that being able to do nothing better than go to one movie represented failure to this once high-achieving patient.)

An important strategy for preventing communication failure is to seek feedback.

Patient: Well, I went to a movie…
Therapist 2: That was good! Were you pleased with yourself? What do you think?
Patient: Not really. It's nothing. I used to be active all day and all night. If the most I can do is go to a stupid movie, I'm in bad shape.
Therapist 2: I think it's good that you got out. It's diversion. It's a good step. *(Instead of arguing and making the situation worse, therapist should have engaged patient by returning to his bad feelings.)*
Therapist 3: So even though you got out and went to a movie, you don't count it as "doing anything?" *(Therapist makes an effort to understand patient before expressing an opinion. None of the therapists in this illustration were in empathic contact with the patient.)*

Therapists need to find opportunities to respond with honest praise. Too much may seem to be contrived or insincere. The healthier the patient (the further toward the expressive pole of the impairment-psychotherapy continuum; see Figure 3–1 in Chapter 3, "Assessment, Case Formulation, and Goal Setting"), the less praise is called for. With the least impaired patients, the therapist should express praise only when it is the socially expected response (e.g., congratulations for accomplishment). Complimenting a patient for persisting with a difficult area in therapy may be useful. The easiest praise comes from the therapist's approval of what the patient is doing. Such praise, however, is actually opinion or judgment. The best praise is reinforcement of the patient's steps toward achieving previously stated goals.

Patient: I took my lithium every day last week.
Therapist 1: Good. *(Judgmental, but appropriately so)*
Therapist 2: Good. That improves your chances for avoiding another episode. *(Reinforces desirable behavior, but still authoritarian)*
Therapist 3: Good. You said you were going to do this—not skip a single dose—and you did it. What do you think? *(Reinforces self-control and discipline; seeks feedback and further engagement)*

Reassurance

Reassurance is a familiar tactic in general medicine. Like praise, reassurance must be honest. The patient must believe that the reassurance is based on an understanding of his or her unique situation. Reassurance that is given before the patient has detailed his or her concerns is likely to be doubted. Furthermore, when the topic pertains to the therapist's domain as an expert, the therapist must limit reassurance to areas in which he or she has expert knowledge. Therapists can reassure a patient about effects and side effects of certain medications, but they cannot reassure a patient about long-term effects of a medication that has just come on the market. Therapists can say, when true, that no side effects have been reported. It is correct to say that most people recover from an acute episode of psychosis within a few weeks or that most people recover from bereavement within a year or so, but it is never correct to say that a treatment is certain to be successful. A therapist can tell a person with schizophrenia that the disease often stops getting worse after some years and later may begin to improve. A physician can reassure a chronic patient that he or she will continue to provide care, because this may matter more than cure. It is never acceptable to offer reassurance that is simply what the patient (or family) wants to hear. If the patient demands reassurance and this reassurance is outside the therapist's expertise, the basis for the reassurance should be made explicit.

> Patient: All day long when my son is in school, I'm sure something bad is going to happen.
> Therapist: You see terrible things on the news, but you know the odds are that nothing bad happens to most people most of the time. *(This is not expert knowledge; it is based on knowledge that comes from general education and popular information.)*

> Patient: I'm having a hard time finding food that isn't genetically modified. It's dangerous. The people in stores don't know, and I get the runaround when I call the 800 numbers.
> Therapist: I know a lot of people are worried about this, but from what I read in the paper, there have been no reports of anything actually happening to anyone. *(Therapist knows only what he reads in the papers.)* It's important to try to keep up with scientific studies about this and to keep in mind that in your total diet, the quantity of foods that you worry about may be relatively small.

The therapist's role, in the face of fearfulness about the unknown, is to teach strategies for dealing with it, not to reassure it away.

Normalizing and universalizing, for most people, are palatable forms of reassurance.

> Patient 1: When my grandmother died, I didn't really feel bad. My mother was so upset, but I wasn't. It made me feel guilty.
> Therapist 1: It's not unusual. Unless there's a very close relationship, children often accept the death of a grandparent as a matter of course. *(Normalizing and possibly absolving)*

Patient 2: When I came out to my parents, my mother wanted to know what she had done wrong, and my father acted like I was a criminal. I still hate them.

Therapist 2: We know that this happens a lot of the time. When your parents were young and forming their knowledge of the world, the experts said that homosexuality was caused by the parents doing something wrong. Also, in those days, homosexuality was classified as a subtype of psychopathic personality. Haven't you come across other gay men who had similar experiences with their parents and who feel the same way about them now? *(Therapist normalizes patient's feelings and encourages understanding rather than expression of feeling.)*

Patient 3: I know I shouldn't be in this program. I'll never understand Lacan.

Therapist 3: Neither will I. *(Using oneself as a standard is risky, but here, therapist assumes she will be seen as a representative educated person and the patient's peer.)*

Adages and maxims are a form of normalizing.

Therapist 1: You can't make your [adult] children like each other! *(Reassurance given as an authority)*

Therapist 2: I don't know of studies, but we know from newspapers, literature, and the Bible that siblings often don't get along. *(Normalizing reassurance given as an educated person)*

Therapist 3: There's a saying: "You can't make your child eat, sleep, or be happy." I guess we could add "or get along with a sibling." *(Normalizing using a maxim)*

Therapist 4: I have never liked my brother either. *(Inappropriate self-disclosure that serves no useful purpose and crosses the boundaries of the professional relationship)*

Reassuring and normalizing must not extend to pathological and non-adaptive behavior or to opportunistic, hostile interactions with others. The objectives of supportive psychotherapy are most effectively advanced when reassurance is coupled with enunciation of a principle or a rule (i.e., teaching).

Patient: Whenever I go anywhere, I have this fear that I'm going to lose control.

Therapist 1: You won't lose control. *(Reassurance as an authority is useful but not as potent as reassurance that reinforces patient's strengths or adaptive skills.)*

Therapist 2: I don't think you will lose control because you have had this fear for a long time and you have always been able to maintain good self-control. *(Reassurance based on patient's history and reinforcement of adaptive behavior)*

Therapist 3: People with social phobia always fear losing control, but actually losing control is not part of the condition. *(Reassurance based on a principle)*

Encouragement

Encouragement also has a major role in general medicine and rehabilitation. Patients with chronic schizophrenia, depression, or a passive-dependent style are often inactive, mentally and physically. The therapist might encourage patients to maintain hygiene, to get exercise, to interact with other people, to be more independent, or to accept the care and concern of others. Rehabilitation requires small steps. Many people discount small steps, seeing each one as of no great importance. Therapy with patients who have disabilities calls for ingenuity in identifying tasks and activities that can be conceptualized as acceptable small steps.

> Patient 1: I don't see why I should waste time in occupational therapy. I'm not going to get a job painting flowerpots.
>
> Therapist 1: Occupational therapy isn't intended to be job training for flowerpot painting. The idea is to allow people to have the experience of staying in one place and completing a task; it's about being able to cope with detail, with structure. It's also, for some people, an opportunity to stop thinking about their psyches or their problems. *(Therapist addresses both the "small steps" element and the diversionary element.)*

> Patient 2: I'm tired of not getting anywhere. My father is willing to pay and I'm going to start college in the fall.
>
> Therapist 2: Before you take such a big step, I'd suggest taking an adult education course at the high school or community college. It wouldn't be all that you want, but it's a low-risk way to see if you can handle regular attendance, pay attention, complete assignments, and feel comfortable with other people. *(Enrolling in a degree program and failing is not effective rehabilitation; it is bad for self-esteem. This intervention might also be categorized as advice.)*

Encouragement is powerful because people want to believe that their efforts will lead to something. Encouragement invokes the world of childhood, where adults do things for the child's benefit; likewise, the therapist can offer specific encouragement that provides a patient with care, compassion, and comfort. *Exhortation* is a more insistent form of encouragement.

> Patient: I'm eating OK, I sleep well, but I can't get going. My apartment's a mess. And they want me to take one of those "welfare" jobs.
>
> Therapist: A demoralized person is convinced his efforts will come to nothing so he doesn't try. The only way out of it, once you are eating and sleeping normally, is to begin doing things. Any kind of work, even beneath your level, can help you to change your perception

and begin to see yourself as a person who can function. Then you can move to something meaningful.

The discussion of encouragement thus far has dealt with only one of the two meanings of the word *encourage*—that is, "to stimulate, to spur." The other meaning is "to give hope." Therapists also use encouragement to give patients hope.

> Patient: All I was able to do last week was go to a movie. I must be in bad shape.
>
> Therapist: One of the worst things about depression is that it makes you unable to even imagine things being better. If you think of something that was good in the past, it's evidence that supports how bad you are now. That's the illness. It may be hard to believe, but these medications usually make a difference and help the depression to lift. For now, do what you can. Does this make any sense?

Skills Building—Adaptive Behavior

Guiding the patient to better adaptive behavior is a major element of the supportive approach, employing the techniques of advice, teaching, and anticipatory guidance. As stated in Chapter 2, "Principles and Mode of Action," direct measures are used. When the patient is significantly impaired, the therapist addresses evidences of impaired ego function. With most patients, the major focus of skills building is interpersonal transactions. Vignettes 2 and 3, featured at the end of this chapter and on the accompanying DVD, illustrate this element of therapy.

Advice and Teaching

Advice and teaching are appropriate in areas where the therapist is professionally expert: adjustment, mental illness, normal human behavior, interpersonal transactions, reasonable living in society, and possibly participation in hierarchical organizations. It is important that the therapist be familiar with the standards and customs in the patient's world. The challenge for the therapist is knowing when to move from giving advice to helping patients learn to find their own way or to find their own sources of advice and information. Offering advice to a dependent person can be gratifying but may deprive the patient of the opportunity to grow.

Ideally, when giving advice, the therapist should include teaching about general principles or methods of problem solving. If the patient senses that the therapist is proposing advice that is not clearly a response to his or her needs, and that instead reflects the therapist's prejudices or convictions, the patient-therapist alliance will be damaged.

Therapist: You should do regular exercise.

Patient: What for?

Therapist 1: Everyone should. Obesity is a major problem in this country. *(Possibly true but presented as a general truth; the patient must infer its relevance.)*

Therapist 2: A number of studies have shown that exercise reduces symptoms of depression. It can reduce the amount of medication needed. *(Includes advice relevant to the patient's condition)*

Advice is meaningful when the patient hears it as pertinent to his or her needs. If the advice is a good idea but not in step with the patient's perceived needs, it is like a commercial or a sermon: possibly true, but not personal—and it may damage the patient-therapist bond. In terms of transference, a patient who hears advice that seems to be boilerplate or praise that is false may experience the comments as a replaying of being dependent on someone who fails to meet his or her needs. Also, every therapist should know which of his or her ideas are based on personal conviction or idiosyncrasy.

Advice about activities of daily living is appropriately given to the seriously impaired, for whom advice may cover any aspect of daily life. It is not given to those who are not impaired, even though it might make their lives better.

Therapist 1: When you get up in the morning, you should get dressed and make your bed. It's important to have a structure and a routine.

Therapist 2: Taking an entry-level job would be a big comedown, but when a person hasn't worked for a long time and doesn't have connections, it's often the only way to get back into the work world. If you later attempt to get back to your old level, it provides evidence to a prospective employer that you have returned to the point where you get to work and do a day's work.

Therapist 3: People who are interested in what you do usually don't want all the details. They may be interested to know that you enjoyed a movie but not want to hear the whole story. Try stopping and noticing whether the other person asks a question that would tell you he wants to know more.

Therapist 1: They offer you free credit, but you're better off not getting into debt. *(Mature wisdom)*

Therapist 2: Let's see if we can work out a strategy about what you should do when you are upset so you don't have to come to the emergency room and say you are suicidal. *(Adaptive skills)*

Therapist 3: I think you should make a plan to begin cleaning up your apartment because it's bad for your self-esteem to be surrounded by evidence of your inability to function. *(Rationale explained)*

Therapist 4: If you don't do something about your apartment, it's possible that someone will make a complaint to the health department. *(Anticipatory guidance that borders on criticism)*

The therapist should not give advice on issues about which the patient can make his or her own decisions. Abstaining from offering such "advice" is one of the distinctions between psychotherapy and social conversation.

> Patient: You know I worry about everything. Do you think it's safe to use my credit card on the Internet? I read that they can steal your identity.
> Therapist: Yes. I've read about that. I think the psychotherapy question is not whether I think it's a good idea, but how you come to a decision when there are different opinions or when you have competing pressures.

The therapist can generally provide advice based on what the patient has reported. However, providing advice based on surmise, even when the patient seeks the advice, is unprofessional.

> Patient: My boyfriend humiliated me in public again yesterday. I screamed at him when we got home, and he said I was too sensitive. I can't take it any more.
> Therapist 1: Tell him that if he does this again, you're leaving. *(Unless therapist is totally aware of the unconscious forces that have kept them together, such advice should be left for family or friends to give. If patient leaves and is then unhappy, she may blame the therapist for giving bad advice.)*
> Therapist 2: Are you able to talk with him about what bothers you at a time when neither of you is angry? *(Implicit advice)*

Teaching is more important than advice. Teaching involves principles, which may be based on technical knowledge or the therapist's position as a rational, informed person who is familiar with the unwritten rule book of life. The therapist's behavior teaches the patient by example. The term *lending ego* was once used as a metaphorical statement that the therapist's model of reasonableness, self-control, and organization was beneficial to the patient.

> Therapist 1: You tend to put up with things until you become furious; then, for example, you scream at people. Dealing with a problem before it becomes extreme is a usually a better approach.
> Therapist 2: Even if you are right, people do not like to be told what to do.

Anticipatory Guidance

Anticipatory guidance, or rehearsal, is a technique that is as useful in supportive psychotherapy as in cognitive-behavioral therapy. The objective is to anticipate potential obstacles to a proposed course of action and then to prepare strategies for dealing with them. For patients who are more impaired, the guidance must be more concrete.

Therapist: What's your plan?

Patient: I'm going to begin reintegrating into society. *(Nonspecific)*

Therapist: What will be your first step? *(Aware that a nonspecific, vague response is not a plan)*

Patient: Well, maybe I'll go to the senior center. My son's wife said she'd drive me and bring me home.

Therapist: Can you think of any problems that could come up?

Patient: She might have to stay late at work.

Therapist: What could you do if that happened?

Patient: It's near the library. I could wait there, I suppose.

Therapist: Good idea. What else? How do you think you will react to being there?

Patient: I wouldn't know anyone.

Therapist: That's hard for almost anyone. What will you do?

Patient: I suppose I could introduce myself to someone who doesn't look too senile.

Therapist: Yes. And maybe you could ask the director or someone in charge to introduce you to a few people. People running these programs appreciate that it's hard for a newcomer. What if you give it a few days and still don't feel good about it?

Anticipatory guidance is especially important with patients who have chronic schizophrenia, because they are especially likely to be apprehensive in new situations, unsure of their ability to grasp social cues, unsure of appropriate responses, fearful of rejection, and unable to maintain prolonged effort. This technique is also important for patients with substance abuse, who often fear rejection and may unwittingly invite it.

Anticipatory guidance may be helpful and supportive in contexts other than rehabilitation.

Patient: I'm seeing my internist next week about this indigestion and weakness.

Therapist: You know, I hope, that you should start with the most distressing symptom rather than with the first things that you noticed, like feeling tired. Are you willing to rehearse what you will say to explain your problem to the doctor?... And if anyone asks, "Do you understand?" and you are not completely sure, say, "Would you go over it again?"

Prevention of relapse is an important supportive psychotherapy objective. The substance abuse literature includes practical lists of topics to discuss with patients to prevent relapse (e.g., Marlatt and Gordon 1985, pp. 71–104). Little adjustment is needed to modify these lists slightly to apply them to the needs of nonaddicted patients with mental illness.

- Identifying high-risk situations and using anticipatory guidance for dealing with them

- Coping with negative emotional states
- Coping with interpersonal conflict
- Coping with social pressure
- Identifying relapse and using anticipatory guidance to deal with it

Reducing and Preventing Anxiety

The supportive psychotherapist intends not only to deal with the patient's overt anxiety, a symptom, but also to prevent the emergence of anxiety. The techniques intended to accomplish these objectives include reassurance and encouragement, which were discussed earlier in this chapter (in the section "Esteem Building"), because anxiety invariably has an adverse affect on esteem. Supporting or strengthening of defenses has been discussed not as a technique, but as a principle or strategy (see Chapter 2, "Principles and Mode of Action"). The structured setting of therapy, the "holding environment" (Winnicott 1965), has an anxiety-reducing effect that contributes to the efficacy of all forms of therapy. In countless ways, the therapist models adaptive, reasonable, and organized behavior and thinking; this modeling is educational and at the same time reassuring and calming.

The therapist should make every effort to avoid the interrogatory style, which involves asking continuous questions and giving little—the style of medical history-taking or the style of a trial attorney cross-examining a witness. To minimize anxiety, the therapist shares his or her agenda with the patient, making clear the reason for questions or topics.

> Therapist 1: I want to ask questions that will test your memory and concentration.
> Therapist 2: Your relationship with your daughter, you said, was a major worry. Is there anything new there?
> Therapist 3: Did you grieve when your father died? Some people have little response and it's all right—but some people who don't have any response have it bottled up inside, and that can be a problem.

Therapist 3 gave a longer explanation. The use of extra words, even excessive words, can provide padding that reduces the impact of an intervention that the patient may find difficult or uncomfortable. The supportive psychotherapist avoids forcing the patient out on a limb, requiring him or her to make a stark response. The following two therapists are trying to obtain the same information, but the second one uses more words.

> Therapist 1: Do you experience sexual stimulation when you see someone being hurt by another person? *(Very blunt)*

Therapist 2: This may seem like an odd question, but it's relevant when someone has a history that involves as much physical conflict as you have had: Do you sometimes experience sexual stimulation in connection with pictures of torture? This could include paintings of martyrs in museums. It's not rare. All those great paintings show that a lot of people have found excuses to portray and look at torture. On the other hand, a person can be involved in a lot of violence and not have this response. *(If patient says "no," he is not in conflict with therapist, because he has been given permission to say "no." If he says "yes," he is in good company.)*

One of the highly regarded interventions enunciated by Pine (1984) is to tell the patient in advance that something might be anxiety producing. This tactic is effective for minimizing the occurrence of anxiety in the treatment.

Therapist: I want to return to a topic that we had to leave once because it upset you. I'd like to know more about what happened when your mother remarried and her husband's children moved in.

The therapist can be even more protective by asking the patient to give permission to go on with an anxiety-provoking topic.

Therapist *[continuing]*: Do you think you can handle talking more about this matter?

Naming the Problem

The patient's sense of control may be enhanced, and thus anxiety minimized, by naming problems. The need for control is one reason why people classify and count things.

Patient: I'm so stupid. I had all those people for dinner, and I didn't allow enough time for the rice to cook, and I thought I was smart to make salad early, but then there wasn't enough room in the refrigerator, and I didn't think to ask everyone if they eat meat. What kind of example am I for my daughter?
Therapist: Sounds like this is just evidence of your organization problem. We have talked about it, and you have made progress. Let's talk about some specific things you might have done differently. *(The objective of "decatastrophizing" is approached by reducing what appears to be a multitude of problems to a single problem with a name.)*

Naming the problem can also be used to meet the familiar medical responsibility of explaining the diagnosis, prognosis, and proposed treatment.

Patient: My mother says I shouldn't lie down so much, but it feels better when I do. I read the ads every week, but the jobs don't pay enough and there's no future. I don't have much money left. It would be great if I won the lottery. There was one job that might have had something, but I would have to commute, and I hate that.

Therapist: This has been going on for a long time. You no longer have signs or symptoms of depression, so the current medication seems right. I think your problem is demoralization. That's a condition in which a person is convinced that her efforts will not succeed, so she does nothing. The only way out is to begin doing things, anything. Small steps can lead to small successes. It's a rehabilitation approach. It affects self-esteem and confidence. *(Therapist names, explains, and gives advice—techniques of supportive psychotherapy)*

Rationalizing and Reframing

Reframing or paraphrasing looks at something in a different light or from a different perspective.

Patient: Everything was going well and then I realized was talking and talking and talking. I've done this so many times. It's as if I have no control.

Therapist: But in the past, you didn't know you were doing it and didn't figure out what had gone wrong until some time later. Now you see it when it happens. That's an advance. *(Reframing—the events are unchanged but given a different emphasis.)*

Patient: I was so stupid. I got a parking ticket, and I could have been back before the meter ran out. I wasn't paying attention.

Therapist: Yeah. That's tough. If you figure it's bound to happen occasionally, you can think of a couple of parking tickets a year as a routine cost of having a car. *(Rationalization—patient benefits from discovering that therapist, who represents the adult world, does not think she is stupid.)*

Rationalization is a powerful tactic for avoiding unpleasant thoughts or feelings.

Patient: My son doesn't come very often.

Therapist: Yes. A lot of young people are completely caught up in work and home. And you manage to get things done without his help. *(Rationalization and encouragement)*

Rationalization is also useful in more expressive psychotherapy.

Patient: My son doesn't come very often.

Therapist: It sounds like you are disappointed, possibly angry. *(Hoping to explore feelings of which patient appears to be unaware)*

The therapist should challenge a patient's defense of rationalization when it is pathological.

> Patient: Yes, I bring things home all the time. My husband says it's junk, but I'm saving a lot of money by not buying new things all the time.
> Therapist: But you told me last time you were here that your husband threatened to leave. Maybe the problem is that you can't control your obsessive-compulsive symptoms. *(Challenging patient's rationalization that she is saving money)*

The challenge in use of these techniques is to avoid sounding fatuous and to avoid argument or contradiction.

> Patient: I feel as bad as ever. I don't think the medication is any good.
> Therapist 1: You look a lot better to me. *(Contradiction—not uncommon in physician-patient discourse)*
> Therapist 2: People who are recovering from depression usually look better and eat better as the medication begins to work, and this happens before they feel better. *(Disagreement, but therapist is conveying expert information that may be useful to patient)*
> Therapist 3: You have to get up and do things. You can't stay in bed all day waiting to feel better. *(Argumentative and not true in every clinical situation)*
> Therapist 4: If you had continued taking the medication as you were supposed to, you wouldn't be in this position. *(Pedantic)*

Often, therapists negate what the patient says thinking that this tactic is useful education. It doesn't help.

> Patient: I was feeling bad. I was thinking about how I used to get up and go to work every day, and I got good pay. I was a somebody.
> Therapist: Well, you have social security now. *(Unempathic reassurance or reframing that misses the point of the patient's situation may have a negative impact on the therapeutic relationship.)*

Expanding Awareness

Clarification, confrontation, and interpretation are useful techniques to make the patient aware of thoughts or feelings of which he or she had not previously been aware.

Clarification

Clarification involves summarizing, paraphrasing, or organizing what the patient has said. Often, clarification simply demonstrates that the therapist is attentive and is processing what he or she hears. Clarification is an awareness-expanding intervention. Both in and outside of psychotherapy, people say things without appreciating the significance of what they have said.

> Patient: I can't get things done. I have to sell the house, but first I have to get some things fixed, and I don't do it. My ex-wife keeps harassing me with court papers about unpaid child support. I think the medication is working, but it takes the edge off my creativity. She's relentless. I'm bipolar. Don't they have to take that into account? My car broke down again, too.
> Therapist: It sounds like you're saying that you're overwhelmed.

Confrontation

As a technical term, *confrontation* does not imply hostility or aggression. Instead, it means bringing to the patient's attention a pattern of behavior, ideas, or feelings that he or she has not recognized or has avoided or defended against. In the following dialogue, which is a continuation of the comments presented in the preceding section, "Clarification," the therapist uses confrontation.

> Patient: I'm living alone in that big house. If I sell it, I can get a smaller place and have money left over, but I just don't do anything. I'm so depressed.
> Therapist: It sounds like you are avoiding doing the one thing that would provide you enough money to pay your bills and give your ex-wife what she wants. *(Therapist knows that depression is a universally used word and that patient who says "I'm depressed" does not necessarily meet the criteria for a depressive disorder.)*

Human beings are frequently unaware of significant feelings. In the early years of psychotherapy practice, often a patient would be unaware of sexual feelings until the psychotherapist helped the patient to become aware of them. Anger also can be outside the patient's awareness. Hidden anger may be directed toward authority figures, people who are more successful, those who are manipulative, or those who are dependent and passive. Anger may be the emotional response to paranoid ideation. The discovery of anger does not always lead to reduction of symptoms or impaired function.

What are some other feelings that are often kept out of awareness? Resentment (e.g., of parents, children, partners, coworkers) is related to anger and is often accompanied by guilt or shame; it is often perceived as a negative emotion. For example, being excessively dependent on another person is often associated with resentment. Grief may be a hidden emotion, especially for individuals who do not grieve the death of someone close. Another example of delayed grief may be in individuals with schizophrenia whose lives have long been disrupted. After reaching stabilization with antipsychotics, they finally may be able to grieve for the years they have lost and the suffering they have caused others. For some individuals, feelings of intimacy and caring are kept out of awareness. Vulnerability scares some people so much that they push it out of mind. The list of avoided feelings can go on and on.

To simply name the feeling and move on is a supportive technique. When exploring a patient's hitherto unexamined feelings and assumptions, the therapist should seek to learn of other instances of whatever has been discovered, talk about the implications of the discovery, understand the basis for it, and ultimately determine what is to be done about it.

Interpretation

There is no agreed-on definition of *interpretation*. Many authors use the term to characterize any proffered explanation of "the meaning of the patient's thoughts or the intent of his behavior" (Othmer and Othmer 1994, p. 87). Others limit the term to a linking of current feelings, thoughts, or behaviors with events of the past or the relationship with the therapist. Linking all of these elements is important for achieving the objectives of expressive psychotherapy. In supportive psychotherapy, however, patient-therapist linkages are generally made only when necessary to avoid disruption of treatment.

> Therapist: You haven't said you disagree with me, but you have found something wrong with every suggestion I have made. From what you have said about your problems at work, it's possible that you do the same thing with other people. *(A linkage between therapist and current behavior; in supportive therapies, such a linkage may help with efforts to improve adaptive skills)*

Insight about historical cause-and-effect relationships is not an objective of the most supportive approaches. However, as stated in Chapter 2, "Principles and Mode of Action," creation of a patient's biography or narrative that makes sense of symptoms and dysfunctions is a useful shared task and often a tactic for reducing anxiety.

Conclusion

Supportive techniques can be enumerated and mastered. With practice, the therapist can apply these techniques in many situations. More lengthy elaboration of techniques can be found in a handful of books. Especially useful are the works by Pinsker (1997), Wachtel (1993), Winston and Winston (2002), Rockland (1989), and Novalis et al. (1993). Guidance about understanding patients can be found in thousands of books on psychodynamics and psychotherapy written in the last 80 years and in literature of the last 500 years.

Vignettes 2 and 3

Vignettes 2 and 3 (presented on the accompanying DVD) are enactments illustrating the spectrum of psychopathology and the associated spectrum of treatment (see Figure 3–1 in Chapter 3, "Assessment, Case Formulation, and Goal Setting"). Vignette 2 illustrates the difficult treatment of an uncooperative patient who has severe, persistent mental illness. Therapy is entirely at the supportive end of the supportive-expressive continuum. Vignette 3 illustrates supportive-expressive treatment to right of the midpoint of the continuum.

> ▶ **Vignette 2: Severe, Persistent Mental Illness in an Uncooperative Patient**

Jerry is a 21-year-old man who was diagnosed with schizoaffective disorder when discharged from the hospital 4 weeks ago. He had been admitted because of self-injury following an argument with his mother. He was referred to the clinic for continuing care. Since completing high school 3 years ago, he has spent most of his time watching TV, playing computer games, or surfing the Internet. He has never had a close relationship.

This is his third visit to the clinic. The therapist has observed that he is grandiose, that his thought processes are characterized by idiosyncratic connections and assumptions, and that he is negativistic. An important supportive measure is honest praise for the patient's efforts. When the patient is negativistic and rejecting, he may perceive a therapist who praises him as an ally of hostile forces. The therapist's immediate objective is that the patient continue in treatment and take the prescribed medication, so her main concern is establishing a therapeutic relationship; she tries to avoid anything that might be taken as criticism and is cautious about praise. She offers advice carefully, with explanations. As often happens in an interview with a new patient who has significant thought process disorder, the therapist at times does not know what the patient is talking about. She does not want to agree with anything unrealistic but at the same time does not want to challenge the patient or ask too many questions.

▶ **Vignette 2: Severe, Persistent Mental Illness in an Uncooperative Patient** *(continued)*

Therapist: So…what's been happening?

Jerry: Not much *(uncommunicative)*. Actually, I just started working. It's a few blocks from where I live.

Therapist: Tell me a little about that. *(Asking for elaboration in general terms; doesn't want to appear demanding)*

Jerry: It's mostly fixing computers. I started yesterday. It's a friend of my mother's.

Therapist: How does it seem after 1 day?

Jerry: It doesn't make any difference *(negativistic and pessimistic)*. It's just like staying at home watching TV. It's really no different.

Therapist: What about the fact that you can earn some money? *(Trying to identify an asset)*

Jerry: I don't care about making money.

Therapist: How many days a week will you work? *(Trying to maintain conversation without seeming confrontational)*

Jerry: Well, there's a movie rental business. I'll look after that and fix computers. Maybe 3 days a week?

Therapist: Oh, so it keeps you busy? *(Neutral facilitator)*

Jerry: It's nothing.

Therapist: I'd say it's too early to know if it will work out, and it's my impression that you don't want to commit yourself. *(Clarification without contradicting)*

Jerry: *[no response]*

Therapist: Is there anything about the job that you might find difficult? *(Looking for opportunity to attempt anticipatory guidance)*

Jerry: I can fix most any computer. It's usually just that someone's screwed them up. *(A positive statement at last)*

Therapist: I heard that the first thing they told every new computer user was that you can't break a computer. *(Still trying to establish dialogue)*

Jerry: They're stupid.

Therapist: So you have a job; it seems like you're quite good at this job *(praise)*—but it doesn't give you any pleasure. Do I understand that correctly? *(Clarification and asking for feedback)*

Jerry: Yeah. It's just like staying home, watching TV. *(Agrees with therapist's perception)*

Therapist: I could go on to another topic, if you'd like. *(Therapist introduces a new topic, "showing the map"—sharing the agenda, asking permission—so that patient will not perceive the questioning to be interrogation.)*

Jerry: *[grunts assent]*

Therapist: Let me ask you this: How are things with you and your mother and your brother?

Jerry: My brother is home from school this week, and my mother has been really getting on my nerves. She lost her job…it puts more pressure on me.

> ▶ **Vignette 2: Severe, Persistent Mental Illness in an Uncooperative Patient** *(continued)*

Therapist: What happened? *(Conversational response; avoiding narrowing focus)*

Jerry: I don't know. She may have a new job. She might start today or tomorrow. Some guy has to call her. *(Patient talks about his mother, not about his long-standing conflicts with her.)*

Therapist: Do you think that she understands how depressed you were when you were in the hospital? *(Trying to maintain focus on patient's relationship with mother)*

Jerry: I don't know. Maybe.

Therapist: Tell me a little bit about the pressure she puts on you. *(Maintaining focus and seeking specifics)*

Jerry: Well, I feel like I have to make money.

Therapist: So—you kind of think she doesn't get it! Kind of like she really doesn't understand…*(Statement is an implied question—a tactic for avoiding direct questions that might be experienced as interrogation.)* And you know, it's funny—some people, they don't really understand mental illness. They think that you can just sort of snap out of it— like it's in your control how you feel. *(An empathic comment and at the same time another implied question)*

Jerry: I don't try to explain. Some people, when I talk, they listen. Other people, no. I don't bother with them. *(Patient is referring to his self-image as an unappreciated teacher.)*

Therapist: Well, you can try again, you never know. *(Vaguely positive; puzzled about patient's shift of subject from mother to "people")*

The patient dismissed the therapist's efforts to reinforce what seemed to be an adaptive step: getting a job. Because the therapist is hopeful that this will help to boost the patient's self-esteem, she attempts to stay with that topic and refrains from approaching the patient's conflict with his mother, even though she knows that this is important.

In the next video segment, the patient makes reference to impairment of sense of self. The therapist deals with it concretely, not naming it as a problem. The therapist's values are in evidence when she suggests that helping people might give him satisfaction at work. She explores the extent of the patient's conviction that making money is wrong—that is, his grandiose rejection of most people's motivation. When the patient accuses his mother of being "negative," the therapist surmises that this is projection and that he is angry because he wants to maintain his dependent relationship with her.

▶ **Vignette 2: Severe, Persistent Mental Illness in an Uncooperative Patient** *(continued)*

Therapist: What would you say about your mood now? *(Avoiding confrontation, therapist elects to start a new line of inquiry—without her usual attention to mutuality.)*

Jerry: About the same.... It's hard to explain. It's sort of a reflection of where I am. If I'm in a positive place, I can be positive. If I'm in a negative place, I'm negative. *(Patient's description suggests a defect in his sense of self, an ego-function deficit.)*

Therapist: How's the work environment? Is that a positive place for you? *(Hoping to find a behavior or an attitude that she can reinforce)*

Jerry: Anyplace you go where the sole purpose is to make money is negative. *(Usual contrary, negative response)*

Therapist: Even if you're helping people? *(Potentially argumentative—therapist hopes to find a way to reinforce the idea of work as adaptive behavior.)*

Jerry: I'm not helping anybody.

Therapist: What if you worked as a volunteer to help people—you wouldn't be making any money. If it wasn't about money, do you think that would be a negative environment? *(Testing internal consistency of patient's thinking)*

Jerry: It would be negative at home. My mother would be angry with me because I wasn't making any money. *(Patient shifts from therapist's question about work environment and returns to criticism of his mother.)* When I was teaching English, I didn't charge anybody. But my mother, it would drive her up the wall if she found out that I wasn't charging anybody.

Therapist: Well, your mother needs money for rent, food for the two of you and your brother, who's still in school. Don't you think that would be helpful? *(Therapist's argumentative question is intended to communicate what she believes are appropriate values.)*

Jerry: It's not that. The only reason she can't get a job is because she's always so negative about everything. Everyone she talks to thinks, "I'm not going to hire this person; this person's going to be a problem."

Therapist: How do you know this? *(Checking on reality testing)*

Jerry: Her tone, the things she says; it's hard to explain. Just the way she talks to people. It gives the impression that she's a negative person. Everything's going to be a problem. That's why she can't get a job. The guy who said he would call her about the job—she called him, and it sounded like she was the boss. The way she acts, it causes her problems. It's not that I'm not helping. It's hard to help someone who doesn't help herself. *(His "helping his mother" and her "helping herself" are not the same, but he uses the words as if they are the same concept; therapist used "help" to mean improving himself.)*

> ▶ **Vignette 2: Severe, Persistent Mental Illness in an Uncooperative Patient** *(continued)*

Therapist: When I suggested that you may be interested in trying to contribute to your family's support, you shifted to talking about what's wrong with your mother *(confrontation, introducing idea of examining unconscious motivation).* When you talk about your own motivations, things sort of get fuzzy and inconsistent *(identifying a problem).*

The therapist wanted to reinforce some aspect of the work situation, but the patient's negative attitude prevailed. He said that his mother was a negative person and because of this had trouble getting a job. Probably, he wants to be supported by her. When the therapist suggested that it would be helpful if he provided money for the family, she used the word *help* to mean "beneficial"; the patient construed *help* to mean improving oneself.

Later, if the therapeutic relationship becomes more solid and the patient becomes able to look at what he is doing, the therapist can try to show him that mixing different meanings of a word (i.e., a thought process disorder, which is an ego-function problem) interferes with understanding and with communication.

Jerry: What I really like to do is analyze things—analyze my life, the places I go, what I do *(grandiose disdain).* The result is always negative. I don't see the point of why people do the things they do.... I see things in a different way. I see things correctly. The way I look at it, nothing I do is really going to change the way things should be. It's like people just decided to live the way they do.

Therapist: Tell me, did something happen? *(Conversational response to the grandiose statement)*

Jerry: Everywhere I go, everyone's trying to make money. Just look at them. There's no point to what they do. They go to work, they come back from work, they go to sleep; the next day they go back to work *(patient's first elaborated response—about his grandiose disdain for people).* There's no point. It's not like they're becoming better at anything; it's not like they're evolving.

Therapist: I wonder if you feel that you can evolve when you're watching TV. *(Deliberately argumentative as an attempt to overcome patient's apparent lack of involvement and to encourage further conversation)*

Jerry *[sighs]*: I'm one man alone, and I can't change anything just being one person. If I try to do something positive with myself, nothing good is going to come of that, because I'm just one person.

> ▶ **Vignette 2: Severe, Persistent Mental Illness
> in an Uncooperative Patient** *(continued)*

Therapist: It sounds like you're really discouraged *(empathic clarification)*. If you could do something really positive that you really
wanted to do, what do you think that would be? *(Hoping to
identify an interest with potential for adaptive action)*

Jerry: If I went to college, I would study philosophy—but then where
would I be? It's not like I can go to an employer and say, "Hire
me; I'm a philosopher." There's no place for people who think
about things these days. *(Therapist missed opportunity to
praise his awareness of reality.)* The patients in the hospital—
they were more willing to listen to me. They realized that they
needed something, and they could get it from me. People on the
outside—they don't want to absorb anything. They're not ready
to listen to anything. So it was better in the hospital. I could talk
to people, and I felt that communication had some purpose.

Therapist: It's hard to change people. *(Tracking, paraphrasing, empathic)*

Jerry: It doesn't change the fact that people need to change.

Therapist: Have you ever thought about the way that you react so perhaps you wouldn't get so upset? *(Challenging maladaptive aspect of patient's position)*

Jerry: I think it's appropriate to be upset.

Therapist: You've given a lot of thought to your situation—perhaps
more than most people—and your conclusion is that maybe you
should do nothing because it all seems hopeless *(praise and
clarification, tracking)*. It doesn't seem to matter whether your
conclusions are correct or not, because the isolation you describe
usually leads to depression *(avoids abstract argument, gives advice based on professional mental health expertise)*.

    Everyone needs activities that are good for them—something
for their self-esteem—teaching, making money, doing something
like that, something that they can feel good about. It doesn't have to
be important in and of itself.... It could just be something that you
like to do. It doesn't have to generate a degree or a career or be the
basis of an education *(gives advice and explains the rationale)*.
And when I say "something that's good for your self-esteem,"
I don't just mean feeling superior. I mean something that really
makes you feel good. Not feeling superior because you can see the
folly in the human condition and feel better than other people *(advice)*. What do you think? *(Solicits feedback)*

Jerry: Sounds like a waste of time. *(Still negativistic)*

Therapist: Well, perhaps you should give it some thought before our
next appointment.

> ▶ **Vignette 2: Severe, Persistent Mental Illness in an Uncooperative Patient** *(continued)*

The therapist stated her position about self-esteem, making every effort to avoid being critical or argumentative. She did not go into the patient's portrayal of himself as the teacher that all the hospital patients wanted to listen to. She explained the rationale behind her advice. Her objective at this point is to establish a relationship based on honesty and openness. In the same visit, she discussed the patient's use of medications, paying attention to possible uncomfortable effects, and to his apparent lack of confidence that anything will help.

> ▶ **Vignette 3: Supportive-Expressive Treatment**

Ann is a 28-year-old woman whose presenting problem was chronic depression. After high school, Ann worked for several years, saved some money, and is now enrolled at a community college. She has a history of relationships that turned sour. Ann described being sensitive to slights and felt she was often treated unfairly, but she did not seem to have ever been delusional or pathologically suspicious. It was noted at the time of initial assessment that she often jumped from one topic to another, and this was thought to be a manifestation of anxiety, not thought disorder. The diagnosis was personality disorder not otherwise specified and depression.

Ann has been attending the clinic for 4 months. She is reasonably well integrated and has the capacity to think about her mental processes, interpersonal relationships, and the patient-therapist relationship. In this video, the therapist responds empathically, praises the patient's efforts, explains her reasons for questions, involves the patient in setting the agenda, praises the patient's efforts, answers questions diraintain focus despite the patient's tendency to jump to other topics, and offers guidance about alternative ways of thinking about what had been perceived as criticism.

Therapist: How have things been going since our last meeting? *(Initial question involves reference to therapeutic relationship.)*

▶ **Vignette 3: Supportive-Expressive Treatment** *(continued)*

Ann: I wasn't so down this week. I got to shop a little bit. But sometimes when I'm there and looking through things, I find it hard to make a decision when there are two or three things I'm looking at *(indecisive)*. And sometimes I realize, "Wow, here I am staring at these things, and people are looking at me and wondering, 'What is she doing?'" *(self-conscious)* But I just kind of push it out of my mind and get over it.

Therapist: That's good. I'm glad you were able to get more done this week *(praise, expressed personally)*. Let me ask you—when you had trouble making a decision when you were shopping, did it lead to any problems? *(Elects to focus on adaptive skills)*

Ann: No. Like I said, I got over it. I was able to sort of move through it. But I guess, since I brought it up, maybe I didn't fully get over it…and that's why I'm talking with you about it. *(Volunteers psychological connection)*

Therapist: What were you buying? I want to understand how this may be interfering with your life. *(Explains reason for question—a demonstration of respect for the patient—good for self-esteem)*

Ann: I was buying gloves, and I was just trying them on, seeing how they looked, if they were warm, how they felt. It wasn't anything as ridiculous as trying to pick out the perfect onion to bring home for dinner. *(Patient is sardonic—evidence of observing ego.)*

Therapist: You said you got over it, and then you said you wouldn't have brought it up if it wasn't a big problem…so you seem to be kind of saying that it is a problem—and that it isn't a problem. So I'm wondering if you think we should talk about this? *(Clarification, then involvement of patient in setting agenda)*

Ann: I think we've talked about it enough. I think we can skip it. I will say that when I got home, I got a call from my mom, and she can really be a pain sometimes. I didn't want to talk to her, but I did for a little bit, and I just told her that I'd been shopping and that I was OK, and I didn't want to give her a full report on my life. I don't know. I don't know if she felt that I was brushing her off. I felt a little bit guilty afterward. *(Sensitive to potential impact of her behavior)*

Therapist: How did you handle her call? *(Initial focus is on action, not feelings.)*

Ann: I was polite. I told her what I'd been doing, that I was shopping, and that I felt OK. I didn't spend much time with her. I hope that was OK for her.

Therapist: It seems like you felt you were brushing her off. Were you rude enough to feel guilty? Or did you feel guilty because you didn't do what she wanted you to do? In other words, you didn't want to talk to her. *(Still focused on action, but adds inquiry about underlying feelings)*

> ▶ **Vignette 3: Supportive-Expressive**
> **Treatment** *(continued)*

Ann: I don't think I was rude. Probably it's how I felt. I just didn't do what she wanted. I didn't speak with her longer or spend more time with her.

Therapist: It sounds like you were asserting your will. *(Emphasis on action)*

Ann: Yeah...yeah, I guess I was.

Therapist: That can sometimes be very difficult. *(Normalizing, empathic)*

Ann: Yeah. My last therapist used to say that it's all right sometimes to say what we mean, and we can have these ideas that might upset us...and as long as we don't act on them, that it's OK. What do you think?

Therapist: I think that's generally true. *(Direct answer to a question)*

Ann: Yeah, I guess. I was thinking [when talking to mother], "I wish you'd just leave me alone. Maybe all this wouldn't have happened—all this trouble that I have in my life—if it wasn't for you." It's *my* life after all. She just really screwed me up when I was a kid.

Therapist: You know, you did say that you weren't rude in that situation *(reinforcing acceptable social behavior)*. How do you feel that you handled yourself? *(Not revisiting childhood, staying with action and self-perception)*

Ann: I think I was good. I don't think she had a clue that I didn't want to talk to her.

Therapist: It sounds like you were pleased with yourself. *(Reinforcing good adaptive action)*

Ann: Yeah, I was. I used to think a lot that things might happen to her, and I'd have these thoughts, and I'd get very, very scared. I'd see my mom getting hit by a car, and all these terrible things happening to her, and I would really think, "Oh, these are going to happen." My last therapist told me that it's really OK—these are just thoughts—and that my thoughts aren't going to make things happen, and I should just relax a little bit about that. And really, my mom wasn't so bad. Maybe I was just too sensitive as a kid. I don't have the same fantasies anymore, but I do get annoyed when she calls. Well, like I said, I went shopping, and I was looking for gloves, I got some food, and I wasn't really feeling down. That's good. I don't know if it's because of the medication. I don't want to believe it's all about the medication. I hope it's also something within me and our therapy. I don't know. I'm trying to get my act together and decide what I want to do in my life.

▶ **Vignette 3: Supportive-Expressive Treatment** *(continued)*

Therapist: OK. You know, you just said a lot of different things. *(Therapist is concerned that patient may have an ego-function problem, i.e., scattered thinking.)* And I think something that's important is to look at one thing at a time. Sometimes when you say a lot of things and you're thinking a lot, it can make you feel more disorganized and more anxious. So I think one thing that's very important is that we kind of take one thing at a time. *(Explains her concern; gives advice)* All the things you said could be very important—you talked a little bit about medication, your relationship with your mother, fears when you were a child. There are a lot of different things, and all of them are important, but perhaps we should talk about each one separately, one at a time.

Ann: OK...so, all I know is that when I finish school, I don't want to live around here anymore. *(Not responding to therapist's teaching)*

Therapist: Do you have any thoughts about what I had said before about your mixing ideas? *(Maintaining focus)*

Ann: Oh, about that? Yeah—I mean, you're probably right. Sometimes I know that I'm doing it.

Therapist: What about what I said before about jumping around in your thoughts as making you feel more tense? Do you think that's accurate? *(Reiterating the point and asking for feedback)*

Ann: Yeah, I think it's possible. And maybe I'll go to Boston. If it's not too big and there's a lot going on...all those schools. Or maybe even to the South.

Therapist: How do you think you're going to decide? *(Focusing on the process of decision making, not the issues being decided)*

Ann: I don't know...I'll flip a coin. Of course it depends on whether I have a boyfriend at the time, I guess.

Therapist: It bothers you that you have trouble with decisions, but from the way you are speaking, it sounds like you are actually able to make decisions just fine. Do you agree? *(Contradicting the patient is generally not supportive, but patient agrees.)*

Ann: Yeah, I guess so. I don't really have to make any decisions now, about where I will go after school. I still have time.

Therapist: Sometimes when you bring up your uncertainty about the future, it's not really a current problem; it's sort of like you're reciting your flaws. Maybe that's a familiar pattern for you, and you're aware of the fact that you are not called on to make a decision right now. *(Naming the problem, possibly challenging a defensive pattern)*

Ann: I don't know. Maybe.

> ▶ **Vignette 3: Supportive-Expressive**
> **Treatment** *(continued)*

Therapist: Sometimes repeating familiar patterns can be a source of comfort *(education about mental process)*. It's important for you that you don't think you've discovered something new every time you do it *(guidance)*.

Ann: OK.

Therapist: Sometimes when you bring up things that you may feel are problematic right now, they may not really be what your main issues are that brought you into treatment. Sometimes what the mind does is to focus on these sorts of things, which makes it easier to not talk about some of the more vital issues. I think that it's sometimes easier to think about these more neutral things. I'm not saying you do this on purpose, but sometimes the mind has a funny way of doing that. What do you think of that? *(Therapist continues education about defensive styles, being excessively wordy to avoid sounding overbearing; then asks for feedback.)*

Ann: I can understand that. Maybe. I've been described as having a "grasshopper mind." *(Patient agrees.)*

Therapist: In some circles, people describe that as charming. And then oftentimes, some people may say that it's a little bit annoying.

The therapist suggested that the patient could alter her tendency toward scattered thinking simply by becoming aware of it, and she provided reasons for being concerned about this behavior. In future sessions, the therapist might, if necessary, look for sources of unconscious anxiety that might play a part in causing this behavior. Whenever the therapist becomes aware of it, the therapist will point it out to the patient and then structure the conversation so that topics are finished before being abandoned. "Say whatever comes to mind" is not the rule for supportive psychotherapy. The therapist praised evidences of adaptive behavior, and she praised the patient's description of her problem, intending to enhance her self-esteem. The therapist did not become involved with the specifics of choices the patient described, choosing instead to discuss the decision-making process.

In the next video segment, the therapist continues with the tentative confrontation that the patient's symptoms served a defensive function and that there may have been an underlying provocative intent behind what she described as a simple question. In each instance, the therapist was tentative to avoid increasing the patient's anxiety or appearing overbearing, because such behavior would be inimical to the patient's self-esteem.

▶ **Vignette 3: Supportive-Expressive
Treatment** *(continued)*

Therapist: How are you doing with school? Are you still able to study?
(Therapist returns to current function with a new topic.)

Ann: Yeah. It's not bad. I get bored sometimes, but it's better than it used to be, definitely. But there is this one instructor in my economics class, and I swear he has it in for me. He asks me questions in class; he's always looking at me. I asked him a question once, and he answered it in a way that showed he thought I was stupid or something. I'm sure it was a put-down.

Therapist: That really sounds unpleasant. You thought you were being put down *(empathic)*. And I think this an important worry— perhaps we can stay with this? *(Therapist wants to maintain focus, and also to involve patient in setting agenda.)*

Ann: Yeah, OK. Since then, I've just kept my mouth shut, and I'll probably pass the final. There's something else that's bothering me. I've been wondering whether it's the medication. I wonder if I'm holding back because I am afraid that more will be expected of me, and I'll begin to be resentful if I can't meet that expectation. Then I might drag my feet and get depressed again. I just don't want that.

Therapist: That's a very complicated idea, and you're quite insightful. You expressed your concerns quite clearly *(praise)*. But something you have to maybe be careful about is almost overintrospecting when you're depressed *(education; tentative, to avoid a challenging approach)*. It's almost like having a pimple that you keep picking at. It can serve to distract you from other issues that are going on, and kind of keep you down and keep you feeling quite bad. What are your thoughts about this?

Ann: It sounds like you're saying that I'm being too sensitive, and I should just cheer up and snap out of it. *(The therapist's educational effort was not successful.)*

Therapist: No...I don't think it's that way—that's superficial. I didn't mean to be sort of superficial, like that. *(Therapist attempts to repair the rupture without going into relational aspects of the miscommunication. Continuation of therapy is not threatened, so transference issues are not discussed.)*

Ann: OK, so what do you mean? I should just...be OK and live in the present? I don't understand.

> **Vignette 3: Supportive-Expressive Treatment** *(continued)*

Therapist: That to me sounds a little bit like a slogan. I don't mean to be giving you slogans, or anything. The point I really want to get across to you is that you feel very depressed, and you are very aware of your thoughts—you're introspective—which can be good, because you have this awareness. But sometimes there's almost too much awareness *(exhortation)*—and there's awareness of negative consequences, and there's kind of a fixation on these negative consequences. There's something called mindfulness *(education)*. And it seems that you are being mindful, in that you are considering your inner world and your thoughts. However, with mindfulness, it's important to kind of leave your thoughts as is: they belong to you—and then sort of let go. And not be too concerned about all the negative consequences and all the what-ifs. Just to sort of step back and be aware of your thoughts without feeling that you have to solve all your problems and act on all your thoughts and worry so much *(expert advice)*.

Ann: Oh, so sort of like, because they're just going to come and go— and I don't need to be so entwined with them? OK, I understand. And thanks for the explanation. I really didn't mean to be disrespectful before.

Therapist: That's OK. You know, I didn't really take it as disrespect *(direct response)*. And if it's OK with you, I'd like to sort of switch gears right now and talk a little bit about what happened in your economics class. *(By pointing out that she is "switching gears," therapist avoids authoritarian style of questioning.)* I know that you had asked a question in class—I was wondering about that. *(Staying with specifics)*

Ann: Yeah, so the question I asked was, "Wouldn't it be more sensible to teach economics as a psychology course?" Then I'd get useful credits for my major. What do you think?

Therapist: I read in the newspaper that some important people in economics are emphasizing the social and psychological aspects *(indicates source of information that is outside professional knowledge)*. But the question that I think is important for us to address is what your intent was when you asked the question in class. I wonder if on some level you were being a little bit provocative with your question? *(Defines the focus of therapy, confrontation)*

▶ **Vignette 3: Supportive-Expressive Treatment** *(continued)*

Ann: Well, I don't think I was trying to be provocative. I thought it was a good idea. Maybe if economics was in psychology, I wouldn't dislike it so much.

Therapist: Sometimes people don't like to be told that what they're doing is wrong *(education about universals of behavior)*. And even though you did put it as a question, it doesn't mean that you weren't making a statement. *(Implied question about adaptive behavior)*

Ann: Yeah, but this is college. Aren't you supposed to be able to say anything, to express yourself, to try new ideas in college?

Therapist: Yes, you're right—it is college. But also you have to be realistic about this. It's a community college. They're hard-working people who are there just like you, just to learn. They're not training graduate scholars. I'm not so sure it's the best place to bring up a deep debate like the one you had mentioned *(teaches about priorities, reinforces current program)*.

Ann: Yeah. I mean, maybe so. I guess it was just getting off topic, or something.

Therapist: Can you buy that? *(Requests feedback)*

Ann: Yeah…I do, I understand.

Therapist: OK…well, I do want to stay with this a little longer *(personalizes question)*. What was your professor's response to this, ah…your question? *(Uses extra words to maintain conversational [not interrogatory] style)*

Ann: He said something like, "That's a novel idea; I don't think they'll do this."

Therapist: It seems like you really didn't like that. And I wonder what you didn't like about that answer?

Ann: It was obviously the word *novel*. You know—"novel"—it sounded very sardonic and sarcastic to me. I don't know.

Therapist: I understand that, but I think it's also important to be realistic and try to understand where the teacher is coming from, too. His priority is to get through the class and to make sure that the material gets taught—not necessarily to engage in a deeper, more philosophical debate.… Does that sound OK? *(Education about the rules of life)*

Ann: Yes, that makes sense.

> ▶ **Vignette 3: Supportive-Expressive**
>   **Treatment** *(continued)*

Because the patient's level of integration places her slightly to the right of center on the psychopathology spectrum, the therapist was able to employ some interventions that are characteristic of expressive-supportive treatment, although the therapist's overall stance continued to be supportive. The therapist addressed mental processes and unconscious motivation, as well as content. The focus was on the patient's verbal coping or adaptive behavior. At times, the therapist padded her statements with extra words to avoid sounding abrupt or challenging.

A few weeks later, the therapist addresses the patient's automatic self-criticism and raises the possibility that role transition, which is one of the main foci of interpersonal therapy, is a factor in the patient's discomfort. The therapist supports adaptive behavior, is empathic and optimistic, and raises the possibility of anticipatory guidance when she speaks of an upcoming date. The therapist supports defensive positions rather than exploring them.

> Ann: Everything is OK, but there is something funny...My English lit
>   class instructor pulled me aside the other day and said, "You
>   know, you're better than your grades. You're always making
>   small mistakes—c'mon, get it together." I understand she was
>   trying to be helpful, but I went home all sad and down and de-
>   pressed again, just beating myself up *(automatic thoughts)*, be-
>   cause I know that I screw up all the time *(exaggeration)*.
>   Everyone has always told me, "Good job; I'm glad that you've
>   decided to go to college, and you didn't stay just working some
>   job." But I don't know—I'm thinking I'm in over my head and
>   that maybe I'm just not going to be able to do it, and I'll find
>   some way to ruin it, especially if I slip back into my depression
>   *(negative thoughts)*. Sometimes I wonder if my mom hadn't
>   been so critical of me, maybe I wouldn't have all this insecurity.

> ▶ **Vignette 3: Supportive-Expressive**
> **Treatment** *(continued)*

Therapist: I'm sorry to hear that you had to go through with this, but perhaps it's not such a catastrophe *(empathic and optimistic response)*. We did talk a few weeks ago about how quick you were to see the negative implications of your teacher's remarks and to start feeling very bad about yourself and very critical of yourself when you looked at his remarks in a certain light *(follow-up on earlier topic)*. And it also seems like in this situation, perhaps you did something similar. You sort of exaggerated the significance of what she said, and you took it very, very personally— and then you started criticizing yourself. And I'm wondering if you were able to connect the insight about yourself when you began this round of worry? *(Establishing that there is one theme and not a multitude of problems)*

Ann: No. I just thought that she was telling me that I make mistakes and that I'm over my head, that it's too much for me. *(Because patient doesn't see connection, therapist decides to move on.)*

Therapist: Well, I have a question that may seem a little bit off topic from what we have been discussing. What would you say is the biggest difference between your current life and the way you lived for the past few years? *(Gently introduces a new topic— role transition)*

Ann: When I was working, I was always doing things. Whatever I did, I knew immediately what to do—whether it was the right thing or the wrong thing. I got paid, and I knew what I was getting paid for. Now that I'm in school, I have no idea. I take a test, I turn in my exam—I get the grade a week later. Everything is so indefinite. It's not very comfortable. They told me not to overdo it, and that I should go along with the plan. And I've been doing that, but if I want something more now, then I feel that I just can't go asking to bring it back. I don't want to look like I'm complaining. I know that school is a good idea. It's been what I've wanted to do all these years when I was unable to do it before, and I had to drop out. It's been my one goal to get back, and now I'm back. But sometimes I just really think that I can't make it. . . . I don't know. I just think, all this time has gone by, and I could have been earning my way since that time that I dropped out.

> ▶ **Vignette 3: Supportive-Expressive Treatment** *(continued)*

Therapist: I think you put it very well *(praise for being articulate)*. And I think a lot of people would find it very difficult adjusting to a new schedule *(normalizing, teaching)*. A transition is a hard thing for a lot of people. You were working, and then you go back to school. And that's a big transition. *(Offering partial explanation for patient's difficulties)* Now, a lot of change has happened, and you discussed a lot of changes. But it's important to remember that sometimes it can take months to really adjust *(education)*. And just because you're having some difficulties initially with the adjustment, doesn't mean it's always going to be that way. It's also to be expected. *(Reassurance)*

Ann: OK…so what do I do about it?

Therapist: Something you can do is that you can remind yourself when you get discouraged that you're doing something that's very hard for a lot of people to do—you're changing your life *(advice)*. And that doesn't mean that college is too hard for you or that you're not up to it—or that perhaps you made the wrong choice. But it's hard and it's normal for it to be hard *(exhortation)*. And as far as not making stupid mistakes, do you have any ideas about what you can do—now that you recognize the problem? *(Reinforces progress; avoids trap of proposing solution to a competent person)*

Ann: I guess I can just try harder.

Therapist: Do you think there is anyone you can turn to for help? *(A question intended as advice to help patient find a solution)*

Ann: I know that in the guidance office, I had seen some material before about how to study more effectively and stuff. It's funny, because when I first saw it, I thought, "How stupid is this?" But maybe I'll just go back and take a look at it again. I think it probably would be helpful.

Therapist: So if you look into it, it may be quite useful; it may actually not be a waste of time. *(Cautiously reinforcing the plan)*

Ann: Yeah…. Remember the guy I told you about before? Well, he called.

Therapist: The one who you met at lunch? *(Demonstrates that she remembers the story)*

Ann: Yeah, yeah. His name is Michael, and we're going to get together this Friday.

Therapist: So, what do you think? *(Open-ended facilitator)*

Ann: I'd like to meet someone nice, and I hope he is. I guess I'll have to tell him that I'm depressed and I take medications. But I probably don't have to tell him that right away. Right?

> ▶ **Vignette 3: Supportive-Expressive**
> **Treatment** *(continued)*

Therapist: That's a good point. Honesty is important; however, the fact that you've been depressed doesn't define you. It's not something you should feel you have to tell him on day one. *(Specific advice)*

Ann: Yeah, but if it's going to be something that turns him off and makes him not like me, I'd rather know at the beginning than before I get too involved with him. Then I'll just be more depressed afterward.

Therapist: That makes sense. As you said, you don't have to tell him right away *(supports adaptive approach)*. Do you have a plan for this date? *(Open-ended question)*

Ann: Do you mean are we going to bed together? I don't know yet.

Therapist: Well, I was being more general. I was more referring to any issues you may have about this meeting that you think perhaps we should talk about? *(Exploring possibility that anticipatory guidance might be helpful)*

Ann: No.

Therapist: OK...during all our meetings, we've talked quite a bit about a lot of things; we've talked about depression, school life, your mother, your past. But there's really been nothing about the men in your life and the past relationships you've had with men. And I know that one of the things you had told me in the beginning is that your depression started at the end of a relationship and that it was quite a nasty breakup. *(Concerned that patient's offhand approach might reflect denial)*

Ann: Yeah, it was.... No, no—there haven't been any more relationships. Most of the guys in school are complete idiots. That being said, I do think I'm ready to move on, and this is only a date. And I'll see how it goes.

Therapist: Well, that sounds very reasonable. Moving on is a good way to put it. *(Responsive praise)*

Ann: I know I haven't spoken about it. I am worried about my ex. He has a new girlfriend, and she was in a car accident. And knowing him, he's probably all involved fixing the car, taking care of her. He doesn't have any money, and I know he can't afford this. He gets way too involved all the time.

Therapist: Well, let me understand this a little bit. He dumped you, right—and now you are worrying about *him*. How do you account for that? *(Considers exploring what may be the defense of reaction formation)*

Ann: Yeah, that's true. I know it doesn't make sense. I was very upset at the time when he dumped me, but I try not to be mad at people for too long. He hasn't done anything recently to make me mad. I don't know...I just try not to be mad at people.

> ▶ **Vignette 3: Supportive-Expressive**
> **Treatment *(continued)***

Therapist: So you're a generous person *(compliment)*. Does your worrying about him affect your ability to do what you want to do? Most people, when someone dumps them, feel quite angry and quite hurt. They may even take pleasure in that person's misfortunes. Do you think it's possible that your concern for him is a mask for your continuing anger about the ending of the relationship? It's funny—that's the way the mind works sometimes. It doesn't have to be that way, and it may *not* be that way, but it is something to think about. *(Use of excess verbiage is padding to avoid seeming challenging or causing anxiety.)*

In this video segment, the therapist was able to praise the patient for her insightful self-descriptions. The therapist instructed the patient about a frequent source of distress that is an area of major concern in interpersonal therapy. The therapist did not elaborate, but plans to return to the topic. The therapist did not offer concrete advice about how the patient might try harder, but rather supported the idea that the patient could develop a solution on her own. If the patient had said she wanted to talk about the upcoming date with a new man, the therapist would have attempted to present several common scenarios to consider how the patient might respond and to explore her fears or likely automatic critical thoughts. Because the patient did not want to talk about the date, the therapist accepted her choice. The therapist suspected that the patient's concern for the well-being of her ex-boyfriend might be reaction formation to mask underlying anger. Had the therapist attempted to go further in this direction, the therapy would be categorized as expressive-supportive; because the therapist did not pursue unconscious feeling, the therapy continued to be supportive-expressive.

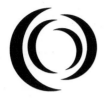

5

General Framework of Supportive Psychotherapy

Indications and Contraindications

Supportive psychotherapy was described for years as the treatment for individuals whom therapists considered unsuitable for expressive therapies—persons who are difficult to treat or for whom expressive techniques are expected to fail (Rosenthal et al. 1999; Winston et al. 1986). From this perspective, supportive psychotherapy was said to be indicated for people who have 1) a predominance of primitive defenses (e.g., projection and denial); 2) an absence of capacity for mutuality and reciprocity, exemplifying an impairment in object relations; 3) an inability to introspect; 4) an inability to recognize others as separate from oneself; 5) inadequate affect regulation, especially in the form of aggression; 6) somatoform problems; and 7) overwhelming anxiety related to issues of separation or individuation (Buckley 1986; Werman 1984).

The findings of the Menninger psychotherapy study, however, indicated that patients treated with supportive psychotherapy made greater than expected gains (compared with patients who received psychoanalytic treatments) and may have achieved lasting character change (Wallerstein 1989). In addition, data support the premise that higher-functioning patients for whom expressive treatments have traditionally been indicated respond just as well to supportive treatment. Their target complaints and psychiatric symptoms diminish (Hellerstein et al. 1998), and they develop a more differentiated and adaptive self because of the interactions in supportive psychotherapy. These changes can be measured as lasting reductions in intensity of patient-rated interpersonal problems after termination of treatment (Rosenthal et al. 1999).

These findings suggest not only that supportive psychotherapy is applicable to patients for whom traditional expressive treatments are not indicated, but also that supportive psychotherapy can be used successfully with a wide spectrum of problems and with higher-functioning patients. Indeed, the most widely used form of psychotherapy is supportive psychotherapy with some expressive elements. Luborsky (1984) and others developed various forms of supportive-expressive psychotherapy that have produced positive results in clinical trials. Supportive psychotherapy may be the best initial approach when psychotherapeutic intervention is being considered (Hellerstein et al. 1994). The therapist should move away from supportive psychotherapy only when there is a positive indication for another specific treatment. In addition to the use of supportive psychotherapy as a starting point in the decision tree for differential psychotherapeutics, there are several indications for which supportive psychotherapy has the best contextual fit and specific efficacy (see also Chapter 8, "Applicability to Special Populations").

Indications

Indications for supportive psychotherapy described in the older literature are essentially a statement of contraindications for treatment at the most expressive pole of the supportive-expressive continuum. These indications for supportive psychotherapy conceptually fall into two groups, which are not really discrete: 1) crisis, which includes acute illnesses that emerge when the patient's defenses are overwhelmed in the context of intense physical or psychological stress; and 2) chronic illness with concomitant impairment of adaptive skills and psychological functions.

Crisis

Persons in whom crisis is an indication for supportive psychotherapy are relatively well-functioning and well-adapted individuals who have become symptomatic in the context of acute, overwhelming, or unusual stress. Under other circumstances, persons in this group might be referred for expressive treatment, because these individuals have good reality testing, a capacity to tolerate and contain affects and impulses, good object relations, an ability to form a working alliance, and some capacity for introspection.

In the case of this group, supportive psychotherapy is usually delivered in an acute-care or episodes-of-care model. For example, a high-functioning patient developed a marked depressive reaction to the change in her body image after a mastectomy. This reaction was accompanied by a loss of self-esteem, a negative attitude toward her work, and problems with social relationships. The patient was able to benefit from an empathic therapist's psychological support, which helped her to begin to grieve the loss of her breast. As she worked through her loss, she began to revise her expectations and plans and gradually returned to the normal routines of her everyday life.

Following are some of the diagnostic and situational indications that fall into the category of crisis.

Acute crisis. Acute crisis is not a diagnosis but rather a general syndromal description for patients whose customary coping skills and defensive structures have been overwhelmed by an (often unexpected) event, resulting in intense anxiety and other symptoms (Dewald 1994). Crisis is the state that individuals experience when they are faced with actual, impending, or possible loss, such as a life-threatening illness, loss of liberty for a criminal offense, loss of personal or public safety (e.g., after the terrorist attacks of September 11, 2001), or loss of a loved one (see Chapter 7, "Crisis Intervention," for a more complete discussion). Supportive techniques may even be implemented in the middle of expressive therapies when there is a crisis for which support is clinically indicated.

Adjustment disorders, in relatively well-compensated people. People in crisis may meet criteria for an adjustment disorder. Adjustment disorders are time limited, lasting no more than 6 months (American Psychiatric Association 2000), and supportive psychotherapy can help a patient to manage uncomfortable feeling states and to shore up or develop coping strategies while the patient and therapist wait for the episode to end. The focus of treatment is 1) to reassure the patient that symptoms are time limited, 2) to reduce stress by clarifying and providing information about what the patient is having difficulty adjusting to, and 3) to support novel coping and problem-solving methods, including environmental change (Misch 2000). At its best, supportive psychotherapy facilitates a more rapid diminution in symptoms and resolution of the episode of illness. In addition, the treatment may help prevent the condition from becoming chronic.

Medical illness. For a large number of medical conditions, supportive psychotherapy is the only treatment recommended. An understanding of the individual's innate defensive, cognitive, and interpersonal styles (i.e., core character and personality) enables the therapist to assist the patient in developing better coping strategies (Bronheim et al. 1998).

Supportive or supportive-expressive psychotherapy has been recommended for or has shown utility in the following areas: reducing pain intensity and interference with normal work, sleep, and enjoyment of life in patients with HIV-related neuropathic pain (Evans et al. 2003); reducing the frequency and impact of stressful events in patients with primary (Hunter et al. 1996) or metastatic breast cancer (Classen et al. 2001); and treating HIV-positive patients with depression (Markowitz et al. 1995), patients with pancreatic cancer (Alter 1996), cancer patients with depression (Massie and Holland 1990) or chronic pain (Thomas and Weiss 2000), and hospitalized patients with somatization disorder (Quality Assurance Project 1985).

Substance use disorders. Early in the treatment of substance dependence, the therapist focuses on development of a therapeutic alliance, both to assist treatment retention and to create a context within which the patient can begin cognitive and motivational work to assist recovery efforts (O'Malley et al. 1992). Kaufman and Reoux (1988) suggested that for patients with substance dependence, expressive therapies (when appropriate) should not commence until the patient has implemented a concrete method of maintaining sobriety, because expressive therapies provoke anxiety that may trigger relapse. (A broader discussion of substance use disorders is found in Chapter 8, "Applicability to Special Populations.")

Acute bereavement. Acute bereavement in patients with poor ego strength will overwhelm their coping skills and defensive operations. These patients generally experience symptoms such as self-reproach, social withdrawal, anxiety and depressive symptoms such as insomnia and anorexia, and an inability to maintain job or interpersonal functioning (Horowitz et al. 1984). Supportive psychotherapy affords the patient an empathic holding environment in which he or she can talk and ventilate about both pain and hostility, have his or her self-esteem directly supported through reassurance and appropriate praise, gain direction for activities of daily living, and reality-test his or her role in the life and death of the deceased. This process supports the use of healthy defensive operations, concrete assistance for routine activities the patient is not able to perform, and appropriate reaching out as a measure against the tendency to remain socially withdrawn (Novalis et al. 1993).

Alexithymia. Patients who are typically characterized as alexithymic demonstrate characteristics that make expressive therapy difficult if not impossible. These characteristics include severe restriction of affect, a seeming lack of capacity for introspection, an inability to articulate feeling states, and a diminished or absent fantasy life (Sifneos 1973, 1975). When these patients become symptomatic because of stressors such as acute medical illness, they may become somatically preoccupied and increasingly dysfunctional, but they remain unable to communicate the effect of the stress on their affective experience. Supportive psychotherapy, through working directly on somatic experiences and personal metaphors, can specifically address alexithymia by helping the patient to recognize, acknowledge, identify, and label emotions, thereby increasing his or her sense of mastery and self-esteem (Misch 2000).

Chronic Illness

Compared with individuals in crisis, patients with chronic mental illness are more traditionally treated with supportive psychotherapy and are more likely to receive longer-term therapy (Drake and Sederer 1986; Kates and Rockland 1994; Werman 1984). Patients in this category typically have a decrease in self-esteem related to deficits in adaptive skills and ego functioning. This group includes not only patients with Axis I disorders that have a chronic or intermittent course, but also patients who have moderate to severe personality disorders and whose idiosyncratic interpersonal styles, adaptive skills, and ego deficits are chronic, pervasive, and maladaptive (Sampson and Weiss 1986). The majority of psychotherapy patients in outpatient psychiatric clinics have probably been treated with dynamically informed supportive psychotherapy.

Some chronic conditions not usually associated with severe mental illness can be damaging to adaptive and psychological functioning and may be helped by supportive psychotherapy. These conditions include later stages of severe medical illness, from which the patient is not expected to recover. Supportive psychotherapy has been shown to assist in reducing suffering and in maintaining self-esteem, adaptive skills, and ego functioning for as long as practicable in patients with chronic illness (e.g., cancer; Thomas and Weiss 2000).

Contraindications

Because supportive psychotherapy is based on the factors common to all psychotherapies, it is contraindicated in relatively few circumstances (Frank 1975; Pinsker et al. 1996). Hellerstein et al. (1994) argued that supportive psychotherapy is the appropriate default approach to psychotherapy and that supportive psychotherapy can be applied over a wide range of psychopathology and situations. Put more plainly, supportive psychotherapy is contraindicated when psychotherapy itself is contraindicated. Fortunately, this list of contraindications is short.

Novalis et al. (1993) suggested that supportive psychotherapy is unlikely to be effective in delirium states, other organic mental disorders, drug intoxication, and later stages of dementia—these are conditions in which any psychotherapy would be expected to fail. Help-rejecting complainers, because they are wedded to the victim role and are not invested in becoming more adaptive, do not make good use of supportive interventions. Instead, these individuals tend to become worse as they confirm that the therapist's goodwill and concrete advice are not useful. Con artists and others who lie or malinger as a matter of course do as poorly in this treatment as in other treatments. Psychopathic individuals, who establish a pattern of pseudomutuality in the therapeutic relationship, either quickly understand the lack of opportunity for real gratification and drop out of treatment, or become focused on attempting to use the relationship to inappropriately gratify real or imagined needs. In the latter case, the therapist experiences the patient as being increasingly needy in order to elicit the therapist's goodwill and expected concrete gain, or the patient becomes coercive to achieve the same goals.

The contraindications for supportive psychotherapy are few. A more formal cognitive-behavioral treatment appears to be more effective than supportive psychotherapy for some conditions, including Tourette's disorder (Wilhelm et al. 2003); acute adolescent depression (Brent et al. 1997), although cognitive-behavioral therapy does not have a better effect on long-term outcome of adolescent depression (Birmaher et al. 2000); panic disorder (Beck et al. 1992); obsessive-compulsive disorder (Foa and Franklin 2002); and bulimia nervosa (le Grange et al. 2007; Walsh et al. 1997). The integration of supportive psychotherapy and cognitive-behavioral therapy is discussed at length by Winston and Winston (2002).

Initiation of Treatment

If the therapist determines that supportive psychotherapy is the treatment of choice, he or she will make that determination during the first session with a patient and is essentially conducting supportive psychotherapy in that session (see Chapter 3, "Assessment, Case Formulation, and Goal Setting"). Supportive psychotherapy is conversational in style and serves as the context for all patient-therapist interactions. In the first session, then, history taking, payment negotiations, interchanges on the rules and conduct of therapy, goal setting, and length-of-treatment discussions are conducted within a supportive framework.

During the initial sessions, the ground rules of supportive psychotherapy should be made explicit, and the therapist needs to obtain the patient's agreement about these ground rules. The therapist may need to temper the message, depending on certain characteristics of the patient, including educational level, ego strength, reality testing, and the context of treatment. The overall idea in creating an unambiguous format for the rules of engagement in supportive psychotherapy is to reduce anxiety by setting clear limits. For example, two clear-cut rules are that 1) no physical aggression and no verbal abuse can be used during sessions and 2) patients should not come for treatment in an intoxicated state.

Office Arrangement

Seating

Seating for supportive psychotherapy is best arranged in a manner that is welcoming, friendly, comfortable, and professional—just like the treatment itself. Thus, the therapist should provide adequate but not harsh lighting, as well as comfortable chairs that are not too close but also not too far apart, so that participants can sit upright and see and hear each other easily. Under these arrangements, the therapist can pick up nuances of verbal tone, facial expression, and body language, all of which are important because supportive psychotherapy relies on a dynamic understanding of the patient. The therapist is sensitive to unconscious communication, even if the therapist does not make that awareness explicit to the patient in the form of confrontation or interpretation. Physical distance, however, can be varied in response to clinical need. For example, respecting the patient's need for distance, the therapist may sit a little farther away from a patient who expresses paranoid ideation. The therapist should not be too far away, however, or the patient's anxiety may increase, because talking face to face with someone for an extended length of time from some distance (e.g., 10 feet) is socially unusual. At other times, the patient-therapist proximity needs to be closer than usual (e.g., when the therapist is conducting supportive psychotherapy by sitting next to a patient who is confined to a hospital bed).

Amenities

In the past, the literature about supportive psychotherapy framed the therapy as a treatment for the most impaired, unpsychologically minded individuals. In this vein, it was suggested that—in contrast to the abstaining, nongratifying position of the therapist in some expressive treatments—the supportive psychotherapist provide, in his or her office, small comforts to the patient in the form of a box of facial tissues on the table or a small plate of cookies or other treats by the door. All psychotherapy should be provided in a humane and respectful fashion in a reasonable setting, and we suggest that this aim can generally be achieved without resorting to feeding the patient to enhance his or her positive image of the therapist. For the most impaired patients, however, the therapist's provision of practical items (e.g., transportation payments) and snacks may help to sustain the therapeutic alliance. Feeding a patient is concretely accommodating, and although it provides a supportive relationship, it is typically reserved for only the lowest-functioning patients. Similarly, gifts from the therapist to the patient are not expressly prohibited if a gift is related to the therapy, such as an informational manual, or if an institutional practice has been developed to supply items of need to the neediest patients (Novalis et al. 1993).

Initiation and Termination of Sessions

The therapist is expected to begin and end sessions on time. This temporal framing of sessions is respectful to both the patient and the psychotherapist. In supportive psychotherapy, the therapist does not focus on occasional lateness; however, when a patient demonstrates a pattern of lateness, the pattern can be explored within the supportive framework. In expressive treatment, the therapist labels the pattern of lateness and adheres to the assumption that the lateness is due to resistance or other unconscious processes. The therapist then encourages the patient's verbalization, with the objective of exploring the resistance and enabling the patient to express his or her wish or feeling, which is generally related to the therapist or therapy. In supportive psychotherapy, the therapist is free to discuss matters of lateness from a practical point of view. Keeping appointments is adaptive behavior, whereas coming late to a meeting that is genuinely in the patient's best interests is not. The therapist can attend to such lateness using a collaborative, problem-solving approach. A pattern of missing sessions can be addressed in the same way.

The following dialogue illustrates a supportive psychotherapy approach to lateness.

> Patient: Sorry, I'm late again. I just don't know—I was sure I gave myself enough time. *[angry]* No matter how I try, I'm always late to everything! I do everything wrong! I should just go home! **(Overinclusive negativism, nihilism, defeatism)**
>
> Therapist: I know it can feel that way, because it's frustrating to have a habit that gets in the way, but bad habits can be broken. *[engaging smile]* Are you sure you do *everything* wrong? If that were the case, you wouldn't have made it here at all today, and you might have forgotten your socks! **(Slogans, humor; challenges the negative self-statements)**

Patient: OK, OK, maybe not everything! *[begrudging smile]* I just hate it when I'm late! It feels like someone's got a fix against me, no matter how hard I try. **(*Esteem-lowering experience of powerlessness, and projection*)**

Therapist: That sure can't make you feel good about yourself. Can we look perhaps at how you decide what time to leave? Sometimes if people anticipate things happening, there's some wiggle room that will be taken up by unforeseen events and leave you enough time to get to an appointment. That would increase your sense of control over things and make you feel better. Want to give it a shot? **(*Empathy and anticipatory guidance*)**

Patient: Sure.

Similarly, a patient may establish a pattern of continuing beyond when the session was scheduled to end, which might have different unconscious motivations, all amenable to discussion in the context of supporting ego function and adaptive skills. With some patients and in certain cases, the therapist might determine that extending the time of a session is therapeutically appropriate. For example, when a patient is unavoidably detained by traffic but is in a crisis, the therapist might choose to give the patient some extra time if the schedule allows or might take the time to briefly connect and reschedule this patient's next appointment if an earlier time is available. Similarly, when patients bring up what Pinsker (1997) called "doorknob issues"—issues brought up as the patient is exiting the session—the therapist is clinically compelled to take some extra minutes to address clinically provocative communications that raise the therapist's acute concern. Concerns about not gratifying the patient's infantile wishes should be entertained but should take second place to reasonableness, which the therapist should always be modeling.

At other times, the therapist might decide not to extend a session, because doing so would support maladaptive, regressive behavior without reasonable clinical or environmental justification. Choosing not to extend a session also models behavior for the patient. The therapist must balance limit setting with promotion of autonomy and independence, part of what Misch (2000) called "being a good parent" in supportive psychotherapy (see Chapter 2, "Principles and Mode of Action"). Sometimes, the therapist must get up, open the door, and firmly show the patient out. Also, the therapist who recognizes that his or her patient continually resists the therapist's efforts to stop on time can choose to cue the patient at intervals about how much time is remaining in the session, thus offering anticipatory guidance. The experienced therapist uses these strategies to wind down a session before time is up, so that patients are not in the middle of a hot topic at the session's end (Pinsker 1997).

Timing and Intensity of Treatment Sessions

The timing and intensity of treatment sessions should be set through patient-therapist agreement, with the proviso that timing and intensity may change on the basis of clinical need, such as when a crisis arises. In expressive treatments, the ideal is to have a constant interval between sessions, which are held at the same time and on the same day of the week. Although the frequency of visits is less fixed in supportive psychotherapy, setting a specific, repeated time to meet tends to reduce anxiety, which is an intention of supportive treatment. Similarly, the length of a session should generally be fixed but be subject to variation when clinically appropriate and when the therapist can accommodate the patient.

Phases of Treatment

Beginning

During the beginning of therapy, the therapist pays a great deal of attention to supporting the formation of a therapeutic alliance, because such an alliance increases the likelihood that the patient will remain in treatment and will have a good outcome (Gunderson et al. 1984; Hartley and Strupp 1983). Over the first few sessions, the therapist should attempt to come to a reasonable understanding of the patient's target complaints and presenting symptoms and to acquire a working knowledge of the patient's general level of ego function and object relatedness, as well as his or her adaptive strengths and deficits. From these data, the therapist synthesizes a case formulation and hypothesizes areas of acute and chronic deficit in defensive operations, adaptive skills, and ego functioning that should be directly addressed through supportive interventions (see Chapter 3, "Assessment, Case Formulation, and Goal Setting"). As the therapist gets to know the patient better, the therapist fine-tunes his or her understanding of the patient's ego functioning and adjusts the intensity of supportive and expressive interventions accordingly. The therapist may require an extended time to develop a clear understanding of the issues of patients who are cognitively impaired because of psychosis, severe obsessive thinking, or mood disorder, or of patients who become flooded with anxiety or dysphoria when focusing on certain details during therapy.

Once the therapist and patient agree on the goals and objectives of therapy (see Chapter 3), the therapist must consider issues of acuity and timing. For example, after a recent psychiatric hospitalization for psychosis, a patient arrives at therapy wanting to talk about whether he should return to college in the fall. The therapist's clinical understanding is that the patient must secure a stable and structured environment in which to live so that he can plan his near-term future appropriately. Without that stability, the patient runs the risk of increased stress, disorganization, and decompensation. However, the patient has brought up neither the imminent loss of his housing nor his plans to deal with that loss. The therapist understands, before the patient does, the need to address issues in a different order.

Allowing the patient to "see the map" before exploring the territory is an important supportive approach that reduces anxiety and emphasizes that therapy is a rational and collaborative process (Rosenthal 2002). The therapist can explain how the topic about to be discussed is specifically connected to self-esteem, to a specified ego function, or to a specified adaptive skill for dealing with psychiatric symptoms or general social interaction. Such explanation is also consistent with motivational interviewing approaches, in that the therapist asks the patient's permission before giving direct advice or prescribing solutions to problems (Rollnick and Miller 1995). However, the therapist must accept that at times, the patient will reject the proposed agenda.

Middle

In supportive psychotherapy, the therapeutic alliance probably functions as a foundation for treatment rather than as the vehicle for change (Hellerstein et al. 1998). Therefore, the therapist continues to monitor the alliance with the patient during the course of treatment and attempts to optimize that alliance by using the same attention he or she used in the initial phase of treatment. This type of therapeutic attunement to the patient contributes to the patient's experience of being understood and supported by the therapist. In the middle phase of therapy, if therapy is proceeding well, the patient begins to accept that the therapist is truly capable of understanding and supporting him or her, and this acceptance can serve as a corrective emotional experience. Positive transference and regard for the therapist are allowed to accumulate in the therapist's account without addressing the alliance, unless it becomes grossly pathological. In supportive treatment, the middle stage can and often does go on indefinitely, especially with patients for whom support helps to maintain adaptive skills or ego functions. During the course of treatment, new, intermediate goals may arise for the patient in the context of life events or increases in adaptive function. An increase in a patient's adaptive function presents an opportunity for the therapist to review goals and to offer praise for meeting goals, as well as an opportunity to offer the patient reassurance and other support for self-esteem regarding goals that have not been accomplished.

In supportive psychotherapy, the therapist has room to use well-structured pychoeducational and skills-building interventions, as well as to encourage the patient to pursue his or her interests and initiatives. At times during the course of treatment, the therapist can present expert knowledge to inform the patient about his or her disorder and its effect on functioning and to increase awareness so that the patient's decisions are better informed. In work with addicted patients, the supportive psychotherapist uses these kinds of educational interventions early and frequently, which may increase patients' motivation for behavioral change. At other times, the patient may arrive at therapy with a pressing agenda in relation to an acute interpersonal conflict or an inner need. In these cases, the supportive therapist will be able to shift the balance from therapist-directed to patient-directed processes, keeping both the patient's goals and the therapist's objectives in mind.

Termination

A formal termination process is not part of supportive psychotherapy. Therapy ends when the goals of treatment have been reached or when the patient elects not to continue. If the therapist believes that the patient's decision to stop is a product of ego-function disturbance (e.g., grandiosity), symptoms (e.g., hopelessness), or faulty adaptive skills (e.g., inability to manage regular visits), the therapist attempts, without arguing, to explore the problem. Even when the therapist has a psychodynamic hypothesis about the patient's motivation, the therapist must balance this hypothesis against the proposition, fundamental to supportive psychotherapy, that the patient is free to stop when he or she wishes. Therapy may also terminate because of external factors, such as relocation or another life event that forces an end to the current scope of work.

At the end of formal treatment, gains are summarized and an agenda is articulated for the patient's continued work without regular visits to the therapist. An important part of concluding treatment is for the patient to reflect on and celebrate important milestones that he or she has achieved (Rosenthal 2002).

Supportive psychotherapy differs from expressive treatment with regard to termination. In the former, the relationship with the therapist is not worked through with the intent of getting the patient to mourn the loss of an important object and to work through ambivalent feelings (Rosenthal 2002). Because constant, positively held objects are frequently too few in the lives of many of the patients in supportive psychotherapy, the therapist does not attempt to get the patient to let go of the relationship with the therapist, which is based in the real relationship rather than in the transference.

In supportive psychotherapy, the analogy of school is useful. The teacher works in the school even when the student is not enrolled in classes; likewise, the therapist continues to work even when a particular patient has moved on from treatment. The patient's treatment can be framed as an organized set of courses, each with a beginning, middle, and end. When the achievement of goals is met, the course of treatment is concluded. However, the student who has a worthwhile experience may return for more schooling (Pinsker and Rosenthal 1988). The patient is always told that he or she should feel free to return if the need arises. The therapist remains available if needed.

Long-Term Versus Brief Psychotherapy

For patients with chronic mental disorders, for whom supportive psychotherapy is primarily aimed at maintaining adaptive and ego functioning, treatment is likely to be framed as an ongoing relationship without a time limit, unless constrained by external factors, such as the patient's financial resources, insurance coverage, or continued-stay criteria in a mental health clinic. At the same time, treatment does not need to go on interminably, if the goals have been met.

Brief therapy is typically indicated when the psychopathology is expected to be time limited, such as when patients have an adjustment disorder or a terminal illness, or when an acute loss or crisis overwhelms a patient's defenses and he or she becomes symptomatic. In supportive psychotherapy, the model of treatment does not focus on character change through emotional insight, so treatment is complete not when core conflicts have been resolved but rather when symptoms have been reduced to comfortable levels or when more competent coping strategies have been developed. A patient may return for more treatment when in a crisis, when the patient needs to shore up failing defensive operations, or when the patient wants to work on something new.

Professional Boundaries

The therapist never takes a turn discussing his or her own needs; rather, the therapist focuses the dialogue with the patient's therapeutic needs in mind. Thus, the style is conversational to reduce awkward, anxiety-provoking silences. The therapist's empathic relatedness allows him or her to know when silence will make the patient withdraw and feel overwhelmed—and when his or her quietness will allow the patient to manifest an important affective response, as the following examples show.

Patient 1 *[after a long pause, a tentative smile]*: Boy, it's been raining non-stop for so long.

Therapist 1: Sure has! Isn't it interesting? Folks often chat about the weather when they're not sure what else they have in common to talk about. It's kind of neat—there's always going to be weather! I wonder if you'd like to talk about how all that rain has affected you, but we can also discuss strategies to talk with people; you told me that's been a problem. *(Normalizing, generalizing, collaborating, anticipatory guidance)*

Patient 2 *[after a long pause, tears well up]*: I can't believe she's really gone.

Therapist 2 *[silent]*: *(Attentive, quiet; empathic concern)*

In expressive treatment, to prevent gratification of the patient's wishes and to promote elaboration of transference material, the therapist typically avoids self-disclosure of any sort. In supportive psychotherapy, the therapist may judiciously disclose personal information to the patient in a purposeful and supportive manner. The paradigmatic model of therapeutic self-disclosure is found in Alcoholics Anonymous and other self-help groups, in which a speaker's lived experience becomes an object lesson for listeners seeking support for their recovery efforts. Many reports on individual behavioral, cognitive, and cognitive-behavioral therapies suggest that deliberate self-disclosure can be clinically useful (Psychopathology Committee of the Group for the Advancement of Psychiatry 2001). Simon (1988) observed that therapists' decisions about deliberate self-disclosure are generally related to several criteria: modeling and educating, promoting the therapeutic alliance, validating reality, and fostering the patient's sense of autonomy. As a rule, self-disclosure by the therapist is appropriate when it is in the interest of the patient's treatment. If self-disclosure is in the therapist's interest (e.g., when it takes the form of ventilating, bragging, complaining, or seductiveness), it is exploitation. Information that is a matter of public record is typically the easiest to reveal in the context of supportive treatment. More private information or personal experience requires more deliberation.

In supportive psychotherapy, the therapist looks for ways to add facilitating comments or interjections that normalize the interaction and to respond to inquiries in a manner that is both appropriate and technically supportive.

Patient *[after a long pause]*: I was thinking, are you married?

Therapist 1 *[if the therapist chooses to answer]*: What are your thoughts about this? *(Traditional expressive psychotherapy–style response)*

Therapist 2: Yes, I am. I noticed you seemed to think a while before you asked me. Was it a little uncomfortable to think of asking me that? *(Empathic concern)*

Patient *[short pause, blushing]*: Yep, thought it might be weird to ask.

Therapist 2: One of the rules here is that you get to speak your mind. It's good you were able to ask me, even though it made you uncomfortable. People who are able to master their fears tend to get more accomplished. *(Praise with modeling of adaptive behavior)*

At times, a patient will ask a question that is annoying or anxiety provoking to the therapist, one that is obviously inappropriate or extremely personal in nature.

Patient: I know you're married, but do you still masturbate?
Therapist: My sexual habits are personal, but we should talk about sexual issues if you are having concerns or problems about sex. *(Clearly reiterating a boundary rule and then offering the patient a chance to discuss sexual concerns)*

Patients with more severe disorders may have difficulty at times differentiating the friendly but professional relationship from friendship. The therapist clarifies and reinforces the boundaries in a nondemeaning way, without being evasive or insincere.

Patient: I've got some Aerosmith tickets! So, we could meet at the box office, and I could give you one. How about that?
Therapist: That's really kind of you. I know that the tickets are special to you, and I want you to understand that I really appreciate that you're thinking of me. It makes me think that our work together is valued by you. But for future reference, I'm not allowed to receive gifts of more than nominal value from my patients. Also, people who have given a lot of thought to these things have decided that it's probably best to keep therapy relationships separate from other kinds of relationships, like friendships, so that nothing interferes.
Patient: Ah, c'mon, doc. It's just a concert ticket! It would be fun.
Therapist 1: You know, I was never much into heavy metal music, didn't like it when I was younger, so I really wouldn't want to go now even if we knew each other under different circumstances. *(Responds truthfully but evasively)*
Therapist 2: I'd prefer to keep our time together focused on our work, which is about getting things done in a very special and professional way, not about friendship. I'm sorry if that's a disappointment. Can we talk about this some more? *(Takes responsibility for the therapeutic boundary but is real and empathic in the relationship)*

Because supportive psychotherapy is more verbally interactive than traditional expressive treatment, and because the therapist has more opportunity to be a real figure in relating to the patient, greater flexibility is allowed for moving traditional boundaries. For example, to normalize what a patient is struggling with during day-to-day functioning after losing a parent, the therapist may empathically disclose his or her own pain and loss of motivation during a state of grieving. With a less abstemious relationship, more opportunities arise for the therapist to use the therapy to gratify his or her own needs and violate the patient's boundaries. Although the repertoire of therapist behavior and speech is broader in supportive psychotherapy, the therapist must always steer clear of the narrow but clear domain of unacceptable therapist behaviors that can exploit patients: sexual contact, borrowing money, or accepting patient favors or information that benefits the therapist (e.g., stock tips, chores, or advice based on nonpublic information).

Conclusion

Supportive psychotherapy is generally indicated as the starting place for a treatment relationship between a therapist and a patient and thus has few contraindications. Other forms of treatment are undertaken only if specifically indicated and only with the patient's agreement. The length and intensity of supportive treatment vary according to a patient's need and motivation, and termination does not require working through ambivalent feelings about the therapist. Treatment is focused on real relationships, including the patient's relationship with the therapist, but the patient-therapist relationship should be discussed only when it becomes problematic. Compared with expressive treatment, supportive psychotherapy allows a broader range of supportive behaviors by the therapist; however, supportive psychotherapy is still constrained by clear guidelines about permissible patient and therapist behavior in the treatment setting.

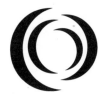

6

The Therapeutic Relationship

Pinsker (1997) and others (Misch 2000; Novalis et al. 1993) described general principles of supportive psychotherapy that are related to the patient-therapist relationship. Some of these principles are listed here and are discussed more fully in this chapter.

1. To help sustain the therapeutic alliance, positive feelings toward and positive transferences to the therapist are generally not a focus in supportive psychotherapy.
2. To anticipate and avoid a disruption in treatment, the therapist is alert to distancing, negative patient responses.
3. When a patient-therapist problem is not resolved through practical discussion, the therapist moves to discussion of the therapeutic relationship.
4. The therapist can modify the patient's distorted perceptions using clarification and confrontation but not interpretation.
5. If indirect means fail to address negative transference or therapeutic impasses, more explicit discussion about the relationship may be warranted.
6. The therapist uses only the amount of expressive technique necessary to address negative transference.
7. The therapeutic alliance may allow the patient to listen to the therapist present material that the patient would not accept from anyone else.
8. When making a statement that the patient will experience as criticism, the therapist at times might have to frame the statement in a palatable or supportive manner or first offer anticipatory guidance.

Transference:
Supportive and Expressive Approaches

Transference refers to the feelings, fantasies, beliefs, assumptions, and experiences concerning the therapist that do not originate in the therapist or in the patient's relationship with the therapist but rather are outgrowths from the patient's earlier relationships, unconsciously displaced onto the therapist. Transference phenomena arise in all therapies, but the role assigned to transference in supportive psychotherapy is different from the role assigned to it in expressive psychotherapy.

In the most expressive psychotherapies and psychoanalysis (one pole of the expressive-supportive psychotherapy continuum described in Chapter 1, "The Concept of Supportive Psychotherapy"), transference phenomena are of pivotal importance for identifying intrapsychic conflicts, and therapeutic gain is ascribed to the emotional working-through of these relationships. The patient-therapist relationship as expressed through transference phenomena is a major area of focus and engagement, whereas the working alliance or real relationship serves as a backdrop from which the patient's observing ego can peer onto the stage (Figure 6–1).

When working at the supportive pole of the supportive-expressive psychotherapy continuum, the dynamically aware therapist recognizes transferences and uses them to guide therapeutic interventions. However, transferences are not generally discussed, unless negative transference threatens to disrupt treatment. The real relationship between the patient and the therapist takes center stage (see "Supportive" diagram in Figure 6–1).

Between the two poles, however, where almost all psychotherapy takes place, a mixture of supportive and expressive approaches to transference material occurs. Supportive and expressive techniques can act as midwives to the emergence of the other approach at appropriate times in a treatment (Gorton 2000), but both the rationale for and content of transference interventions by the therapist are different in supportive and expressive treatments.

Supportive therapists track transference material but address it only when necessary. Focusing on positive transference material in supportive psychotherapy is generally unnecessary.

> Patient: Doctor, you always give me the right advice, even when I'm not on the ball or I have some wrong idea. How'd you get so smart?
> Therapist: Thanks, but I can't take all the credit. I had good teachers, and I have learned a lot of effective principles from working with patients. *(Accepts the positive statement but modulates it slightly with reality testing)*

Negative transference is more typically a focus in supportive psychotherapy, because such transference can be a threat to the integrity of the treatment and normally adds to the patient's suffering when acted on outside the treatment setting. In supportive and supportive-expressive psychotherapy, the therapist clarifies often and confronts at intervals, but inter-

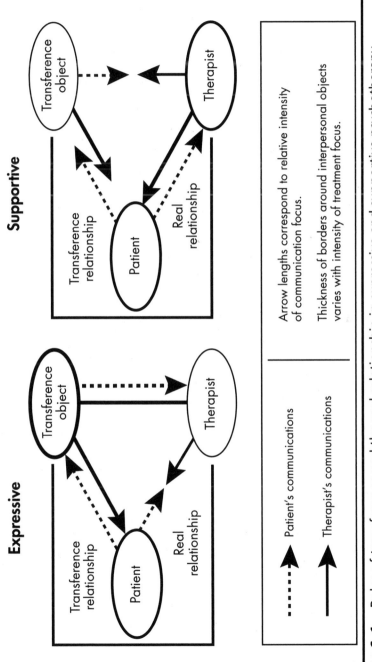

Figure 6–1. Roles of transference and the real relationship in expressive and supportive psychotherapy.

Source. Adapted from Pinsker et al. 1991.

prets infrequently. The therapist's interventions assist the patient in recognizing and addressing maladaptive behavioral or construal patterns that are reflected in behavior with the therapist; a goal of these interventions is to increase the patient's self-esteem and adaptive functioning. The patient's behavior with the therapist in supportive treatment is understood to be illustrative of the patient's behavior with others.

In expressive treatment, transference clarification and interpretation are important interventions. In this treatment, the patient's characterological and core neurotic defenses are often expressed through positive and negative transference phenomena. The therapist's transference interpretations and clarifications assist the patient in gaining insight and working through unconscious conflicts; a goal of these interventions is character change. In expressive therapy, relationships between the patient and other people are used to illuminate the central patient-therapist relationship.

The content of the therapist's transference interpretation also differs in expressive versus supportive modes. The precision and comprehensiveness of an interpretation may vary, depending on the level of the patient's object relations and defensive functioning, the patient's progress in treatment, and the strength of the therapeutic alliance. Interventions often have more of the quality of clarifications and confrontations than of interpretations in the strict sense. Typically, the healthier a patient is on the continuum of psychopathology, the better he or she will tolerate a precise and comprehensive interpretation without damaging the therapeutic alliance. However, the therapist can present interpretive ideas in a supportive manner (Winston et al. 1986). In working with patients who are more impaired on the continuum, the therapist rarely makes full interpretations but may make incomplete interpretations (leaving out genetic references and generalizing [Pinsker et al. 1991]) or inexact interpretations (diluting infantile fears with other plausible explanations [Glover 1931].

> Therapist 1: So, keeping your room messy is a way for you to in a sense be independent and to do things in your own way in your own space, as compared with how it is at work, where everything must be annoyingly in its place and on time. Is there a downside? *(Supports self-esteem, makes a connection to angry feeling, contrasts patient's style with real-world expectation, opens a dialogue on adaptive skills)*

In the midst of an expressive treatment, the therapist might use interpretation.

> Therapist 2: So, keeping your room messy is a way of setting things up, hoping your mother cleans it up. She's supposed to make it OK, and you get anxious about it. Then you become enraged and feel you have little control. *(Makes a primary connection to a genetic figure*

and to the role of aggression in staving off anxiety when depen-
dency needs are not met)

The Therapeutic Alliance

In supportive and supportive-expressive psychotherapies—for example, brief supportive psychotherapy (Hellerstein et al. 1998), brief adaptive psychotherapy (Pollack et al. 1991), and supportive-expressive psychotherapy (Luborsky 1984)—an early and strong therapeutic alliance (which is reflective of the real relationship) is predictive of positive outcome in treatment and thus is a major focus of treatment (Westerman et al. 1995; Winston and Winston 2002).

In the early days of psychoanalysis, Freud acknowledged that transference included a personal relationship with the patient, which he called "rapport" or "unobjectionable positive transference." He considered this relationship necessary to maintain the motivation needed to collaborate effectively and therefore maintained that the relationship was not to be interpreted (Gill and Muslin 1976; Safran and Muran 2000). This view is the earliest evidence of a principle within psychodynamic treatments for managing a strong therapeutic alliance, and Freud's view provides a basis for not interpreting positive transference in supportive psychotherapy. As the concept of the therapeutic alliance began to develop, the focus shifted to the working relationship between the patient and therapist and began to be framed as a "working alliance," with elements of the real relationship that were separate from the transference (Greenson 1965, 1967; Zetzel 1956).

Current conceptions of the alliance are broader and seem a commonsense fit with the construct of supportive psychotherapy. The strength of the therapeutic alliance hinges on the extent of patient-therapist agreement on therapeutic tasks and goals, the patient's capacity to perform the therapeutic work, the therapist's empathic relatedness and involvement, and the robustness of the affective bond between patient and therapist (Bordin 1979; Gaston 1990).

The therapeutic alliance is most likely the therapeutic foundation for change rather than the vehicle for change, as hypothesized for more expressive treatments (Gaston 1990; Hellerstein et al. 1998; Horvath and Symonds 1991). Therefore, the therapist fosters the alliance through active measures, acting as a good role model and "parent" and being tolerant and nonjudgmental (Misch 2000). Direct measures that support the patient's self-esteem support the therapeutic alliance, which has a basis in the real relationship. The patient may have a fantasy about the therapist's capacities (transference), but the therapist is actively engaged with the patient in a real relationship and is providing what is often concrete help to the patient.

Misalliance: Recognition and Repair

To promote effective psychotherapy, the therapist must pay attention to rifts in the patient-therapist alliance and make concerted efforts to repair them. In supportive treatment, because the therapist is active, he or she has greater opportunity to say the wrong thing and to step on the patient's toes. At the same time, supportive psychotherapy does not emphasize exploration of conflict, in an attempt to avoid anxiety that might interfere with a positive alliance. In the event of a rupture, the supportive psychotherapist has ample opportunity, as well as a breadth of strategies, to intervene effectively. Less constraint is placed on the ways in which the therapist might communicate his or her distress at being misunderstood by the patient, as well as sincere regret at having unwittingly impugned or patronized the patient or having raised a subject that the patient found intrusive, anxiety provoking, or simply unpalatable. Generally, when the therapist anticipates or notices a misalliance, he or she uses standard supportive techniques to address it, because supportive measures are the first line of repair for ruptures in the alliance (Bond et al. 1998). The therapist attempts to address the problem practically, in the context of the current situation, before moving to symbolic or transference issues (Pinsker 1997). The following vignette demonstrates how a therapist addressed a misalliance (see Vignette 4 on the DVD).

> ▶ **Vignette 4:**
> **Addressing a Misalliance**

The patient is a 35-year-old single woman, a computer engineer, who has been treated successfully with antidepressants for major depression, with resulting increased energy, libido, and concentration. She is typically passive and compliant in her interpersonal dealings and has had long-term difficulty communicating directly what she wants in social and intimate relationships. She has had several serious long-term relationships with men that demonstrate a pattern of her being too accommodating, with a resultant loss of self-esteem and a buildup of resentment. Because she is passive and dependent, she has often tolerated a significant lack of reciprocity in her relationships, frequently reporting having been "bossed around," yet has stayed in them even when she was no longer happy. Her current boyfriend of 8 months, another computer engineer, is irritable, perfectionistic, and critical, frequently blaming the patient when things don't go as planned. When her needs and desires are frustrated, she becomes sullen, sarcastic, and full of self-recrimination, which further lowers her self-esteem.

> ▶ **Vignette 4:**
> **Addressing a Misalliance (*continued*)**

The therapist has been trying over several months to support the patient in "finding her voice" so that she might be better able to navigate getting her needs served in the current relationship and "make it work." The therapist is using a model with the patient of what he deems to be adult behavior in a committed relationship.

Patient: I don't know why I'm here *[sullen]*.

Therapist: Could you clarify what you mean?

Patient: All we do is argue, and he never owns up to anything. Just asks me questions, expects me to do whatever he wants, and never tells me what he really thinks. I try to be reasonable, but it's always his way, and it's always my fault. Now it looks like it's over—the relationship's just over!

Therapist: I still don't understand. You've described this pattern to me many times before: having a good time, followed by struggling with your boyfriend, and then thinking that it is over.

Patient: That's right.

Therapist: OK, but I'm unclear as to what you mean by your statement that you don't know why you're here. (**Attempts, through clarification and confrontation, to get the patient to become more specific**)

Patient: What good is this? I talk and talk here, and now another relationship is blowing up because I can't sustain it. I try to do the right thing, and it doesn't make any difference. I can't do it right enough.

Therapist: And...

Patient: So, I don't know why I'm here. (**Again, lodges a complaint about the treatment not giving her what she needs, despite her doing what she believes she is asked**)

Therapist: We look at these patterns in your relationship so that you can learn ways to change them or learn how to do things differently, which can improve your relationship and your self-esteem. (**Indirectly attempts to strengthen the therapeutic alliance by reiterating common goals**)

Patient: Big words.

Therapist: I thought I was being clear in talking to you about this, but perhaps I'm missing something.

Patient: *[frowns and raises her shoulders]*

Therapist: You've been working hard the past few months in our work together, so that you might be better able to get more out of what you want from this relationship. (**Praise for hard work in therapy**)

Patient: See, you're just like him. I try to do things right, and it still doesn't work out *[looks down, sullen]*. *(States that therapist behaves similarly to boyfriend with similar impact)*

Therapist: Are you saying that you see me as having expectations of you here and that when you try to do the right thing, it doesn't seem to work out, and you still feel low and frustrated? *(Clarifies)*

Patient *[nods her head and frowns]*: Yes.

Therapist: I see. I've been supporting you in working on this relationship, in "doing the right thing," but I think you're stuck in a process that has you feeling one down, and not just with him, but here too. And it's not good for you and it's not good for your self-esteem. I can own up to that, and I want to be better able to assist you in our work together. *(Therapist "owns up" to supporting the patient's staying in the relationship, which the patient feels diminishes her autonomy, as the relationship with the boyfriend reduces her self-esteem.)* If there is a style that I'm using that is actually lowering your self-esteem, I'll consider changing it for something that works better for you. *(Directly allies with the patient, demonstrates responsive, adult behavior)*

Patient: You can do that? *[looks up at the therapist, alert]*

Therapist: Yes, of course.

Patient: That's different from him. *(Recognizes a component of the real relationship with the therapist as contrasted with transference or boyfriend)*

Therapist: In the past I have supported your attempts on working on this relationship with this man, but you continue to have these powerful disputes where you end up feeling disempowered and blamed. While I can understand your disappointment and sadness in ending it, I do think that you are correct. Staying with this man is damaging to your self-esteem. Here I've been trying to help you to stay and figure out a way to work it out because I thought I had your best interests in mind, but now I think that you know better about your own life. I'm sorry I didn't catch on earlier. Where do we go from here? *(At times, the therapist may have to change his or her position, as people normally do when talking with someone who is becoming angry or distant.)*

> **Vignette 4:**
> **Addressing a Misalliance** *(continued)*

The patient's talk about the relationship blowing up is also a transferential statement about her experience of the therapy and the therapist. Up to this point, she expressed herself as helpless to reveal to him that the strategy was not working and that she was feeling worse. When the therapist discloses to the patient that he has been using a model that sets up the expectation that she "do the right thing," he sidesteps the transferential bind he may have put himself in with respect to this patient. She begins to experience him differently, such that the alliance is strengthened and the patient feels that she has been heard.

Resistance

Many therapists might say that the concept of resistance is relevant only to the expressive element of therapy, in which uncovering is essential. However, some of these therapists use the term *resistance* broadly to signify any patient-produced obstacle to achieving the goals of therapy. In this sense, resistance may be characterized as the nearly universal out-of-awareness fear of new ways and the tendency to cling to familiar patterns even when they are maladaptive. Because supportive treatment aims to support adaptive defenses and build self-esteem, the therapist's strategy in relation to resistance is to increase the patient's motivation for action through encouraging problem solving and the learning of new adaptive skills.

Another obstacle to treatment is a traitlike disposition to avoid painful affects, which can interfere with treatment even when the therapist makes every effort to mitigate discomfort or anxiety. In examining the traitlike components of resistance, Beutler et al. (2002b) presented evidence from several studies that measures of patient characteristics typically associated with trait resistance—such as defensiveness, anger, impulsivity, and direct avoidance—are negatively correlated with psychotherapy outcomes. These findings have direct relevance for supportive psychotherapy: patients with high levels of trait resistance tend to have better outcomes with dynamic nondirective, self-directed, or relationship-oriented therapies (e.g., supportive-expressive psychotherapies) than with structured cognitive or behavioral treatments (Beutler et al. 2002b).

"Joining the Resistance"

Supportive treatment aims to support defenses unless they are maladaptive. Again, a primary principle in supportive psychotherapy is to support the therapeutic alliance. When a patient is resistant to looking at dysfunctional patterns, the fact that the therapist reflects the patient's despair and hopelessness or empathizes with his or her tough life or work situation might give the patient a strong sense of being understood and thus increase his or her willingness to work in therapy (Messer 2002). Supportive psychotherapy can provide, without coercion, an active empathic environment and reinforcement of the patient's stated goals.

In supportive-expressive treatment, when a patient is struggling with recognizing his or her own feelings or impulses, the therapist can follow the patient's lead and make empathic statements about how difficult and anxiety provoking it is to reveal oneself (Messer 2002).

> Patient: Mom was usually pretty good about getting to games on time, but Dad used to show up sometimes…usually after the fact. He was always really busy…*[looks sad]* and we got along…OK. *[pause]* Hey, you know why I was late today? The cabdriver on the way here—the stupid guy couldn't drive worth a damn! What a joke. How'd he get a license?
>
> Therapist: It seems that it's making you anxious to focus on how you really feel toward your father.
>
> Patient: This is hard. I don't think I can do this *[tearing]*. What if I can't do this? **(Increased anxiety, self-doubt)**
>
> Therapist: Talking about this kind of difficult stuff makes people anxious, but they get through it in psychotherapy. I want you to know that your pursuing it and revealing it here takes courage. I think you're clearly capable of doing it. I wouldn't support your looking at your feelings toward your father if I thought you weren't capable. **(Empathy, normalization, accurate praise, reassurance)**

Reducing Anxiety to Facilitate Discussion

Showing the patient a map before exploring the territory reiterates that the engagement is collaborative and centers around agreed-on goals. Anxiety is often diminished when the patient becomes cognitively aware of what is being offered for discussion.

> Patient: Sorry I'm late. I started out with plenty of time, but some things came up, and before I knew it, it was 20 after.
>
> Therapist: Have you noticed that over the last few weeks, you've come into the session about 20 minutes before our time is up? I feel bad that you may not be getting what you are paying for. Could we talk about it? **(With other patients, the therapist might be uncertain if consistent lateness is related to feelings about the therapy or the**

therapist or if it is due to deficits in ego function or adaptive skills. In this case, the therapist knows from earlier sessions that the patient's lateness is related to the therapist.)

Patient: Sure, but I just had stuff to do, and I lost track of the time. *(Rationalizes, deflects, plays the lateness off as a result of making more important choices)*

Therapist: In psychotherapy, when someone creates a pattern of somehow getting to the session with only a little time left, it may mean that there is something the person is wrestling with inside that is showing up in this behavior pattern. People do well with looking at what's inside them, exploring it, though sometimes it brings up uncomfortable emotions. I'm happy to explore it with you if you are interested. It might be helpful. *(Clarifies, confronts, normalizes, offers guidance about the cost of exploring this issue)*

Patient: It's not just here, doc. I'm late for everything *[sheepish grin]. (Generalizes away from the therapy situation but owns the pattern)*

Therapist: So, as a bonus, if we can explore that pattern here, maybe you can learn a skill or a principle that helps you to get along better out there. Is that something you'd be interested in? *(Supports motivation, enlists collaboration)*

Patient: Sure.

Reframing Resistance as Healthy Self-Assertion

The therapist can address opposition to his or her efforts by framing it as a healthy function of the patient's need for control and self-assertion; the therapist may reduce the resistance by becoming more accepting and authentic (Beutler et al. 2002a).

Patient: I didn't ask my mom to enroll me for the spring semester…like we talked about last time. I decided to put it off until the fall. I'm just not ready to do that yet. Are you angry?

Therapist: It's good that you know your own mind and can make a definitive decision. You must feel some relief about taking a stand. I'm not angry, because I don't get to make the decisions about your life, only to look at the decisions together with you and try to help you with how you make them.

Dealing With Distance and Withdrawal

Patients frequently demonstrate resistance in sessions through withdrawal and noninteraction. Because the therapist's verbal responsiveness is a characteristic of supportive psychotherapy, the therapist does not wait for things to unfold if the patient is silent. Doing so supports resistance and may increase the patient's anxiety. In supportive psychotherapy, when the patient is silent or unresponsive, the therapist selects an issue for attention. The issue may be directly related to the patient's lack of verbal engagement, which the therapist might choose to address indirectly. Alternatively, the therapist might switch to another topic entirely.

> Patient: Hello again. *[sits down]* I don't really have much to talk about today. *[sits quietly, looking at the therapist blankly]*
>
> Therapist 1 *[warmly]*: It's good to see you again. So, can we get back to the topic you were discussing with me before I left on vacation? You were describing how hard it was to follow through on asking for a transfer at work and how those "Why bother?" thoughts were getting in your way. *(The therapist picks up the patient's topic from before the therapist's absence, reconnecting with the patient and supporting the patient's self-esteem by showing that the patient was important enough to the therapist for the therapist to remember the issue. This approach focuses indirectly on the patient's distancing maneuvers and sidesteps what the therapist assumes are the patient's negative emotions about the therapist's absence and increased anxiety about revealing them.)*
>
> Therapist 2: Hello. It's good to see you again. Well, it's been 3 weeks since our last session. Although I had someone covering for emergencies, it's not the same as coming for therapy.
>
> Patient: That's right. *[looks at the therapist less blankly]* *(Engages a bit, reinforces the therapist's coming in closer)*
>
> Therapist 2: Sometimes, when people say they don't have anything on their mind or much to talk about, they actually do but aren't quite sure whether to or how to say something. Patients often find themselves in that situation when their therapists come back after a vacation. *(Clarifies the situation but generalizes away from the specifics of the patient and the therapist before confronting the patient's denial and withdrawal)*

The therapist must be alert to distancing negative responses and be able to anticipate and avoid a disruption in treatment. Not addressing misalliance may lead to a treatment disruption. The therapist must decide whether the situation requires intervention through confrontation or whether indirect means will suffice. The therapist must always evaluate, through introspection, and determine that he or she is not becoming involved in a countertransference enactment (Robbins 2000).

Countertransference

As aptly stated by Clever and Tulsky (2002), "Asking patients to tell us what they want potentially opens an imagined Pandora's box of outrageous requests, and it requires energy both to negotiate this tactfully and to manage the countertransference such negotiation produces in ourselves" (p. 893).

Defining Countertransference

In considering countertransference, the therapist must make a distinction between 1) emotional reactions to a patient's behavior that are due to the therapist's issues and 2) emotional reactions that are the therapist's response to the patient's unconscious attempt to provoke a reaction, which might be a manifestation of transference, coming from the patient's internal world (Messer 2002).

The first type of countertransference is what has been described as the narrow or classical view of countertransference, essentially the therapist's transference to the patient (Gabbard 2001). A broader definition of countertransference includes the real relationship, consisting of reactions most people would have to the patient, as determined by moment-to-moment patient behavior in the therapeutic relationship. On a related note, when the therapist is lacking in expertise or when the type of therapy is not helpful for the patient or problem, the therapist might mistakenly identify his or her bad feelings about the patient and treatment as countertransference, or the therapist might misperceive the problem as the patient's resistance. The therapist makes an attribution that the patient is being resistant, but actually the therapist or treatment is not effective.

Because we describe supportive psychotherapy as a dynamically informed treatment, the second or broader view of countertransference has a place in our discussion of technical work with patients. This view is that emotional reactions of the therapist to the patient represent useful information related to the patient's inner world and unconscious processes (Gabbard 2001). Currently, many psychoanalytic theorists from varying perspectives form a consensus view that countertransference is a transactional construct, affected by what the therapist brings to the situation as well as by what the patient projects (Gabbard 2001; Kiesler 2001). A discussion of therapist transference is beyond the scope of this chapter, but it is incumbent on the therapist to attempt to distinguish his or her own feelings from those provoked by the patient, or in the case of projective identification, those that arise in the patient.

Supportive psychotherapy aims to improve adaptive skills. Maladaptive behavior patterns in the patient's real life frequently manifest as countertransference elicitations in the therapy session. When the therapist recognizes that his or her reactions to the patient are the same as everyone else's reactions, sharing this awareness with the patient may be useful in framing practical interventions to assist the patient with better interpersonal adaptation. The therapist must be aware, however, that his or her intent to self-disclose feelings toward the patient could represent the therapist's own needs, not the requirements of the therapeutic situation. Such an awareness is more important in supportive psychotherapy, in which the flow of dialogue is conversational, than in expressive treatment, in which the therapist may at times abstain from responding. Gelso et al. (1995, 2002) demonstrated that better countertransference management correlated positively with better outcome in brief therapy (consisting of 12 sessions).

The therapist in the following dialogue recognizes the patient's maladaptive behavior pattern.

> Patient: Everyone always blows me off. I try to be nice—you know...join in, tell stories and stuff—then I see them look at each other, and they throw it in my face, and they make excuses and leave. Like they're so cool. That Andy—he's a piece of work, and I told him so.
>
> Therapist: It must be hard to try joining in and be rejected like that. *(Empathic)*
>
> Patient: Stop talking down to me. Jeez, you shrinks always act like you're Mother Teresa, but she didn't take the money for herself, did she? *(Feels impugned, attacks by questioning the therapist's motives)*
>
> Therapist: Hmm. It sounds like how you are being here with me is how you've described interacting with Andy and Fred at work. I'm finding my temperature rising with your criticisms of me, and I can't help but wonder if you get the guys at work to feel the same way— except I won't act on my feelings the way that they do. I'll continue to sit and talk with you; I won't make excuses and leave. *(Modulated confrontation, drawing of parallels. The therapist restates her commitment to the process and offers disconfirmation of the patient's expected rejection in spite of the pressure to reject the patient.)*
>
> Patient: Oh, sure! Now you're saying it's my fault you're angry? *(Continues the verbal assault, feels criticized anyway)*
>
> Therapist: I think if we get into an argument, I won't be doing my job of being helpful to you, and you'll keep feeling put down. No, what I'm asking you to do is to see if there's a pattern here that we can work on to help you to get along better with people, because you've told me you would like that. *(Clarifies, does not get pulled into acting out of countertransference feeling but uses the countertransference knowledge productively by recommitting to the work, focusing on the alliance in spite of heightened feelings, and reinforcing the patient's treatment goal)*

From the vantage point of interpersonal communication theory, Kiesler (2001) described effective feedback of countertransference feelings as applying the principle that disclosing metaphors or fantasies has the least threatening effect, compared with direct feelings or tendencies toward action. This principle is highly consistent with supportive psychotherapy approaches, in which it is safer, more respectful, and more protective of the therapeutic alliance to say, "I'm finding my temperature rising," than to say, "I'm so angry, I feel like punching you out." The therapist's modulated expression of countertransference feeling not only offers disconfirmation of the patient's maladaptive construal style but also models adult restraint and containment (but not denial) of affect. The therapist who responds to the patient's hostility in a complementarily hostile way is arguing. Besides being bad supportive technique, a therapist's hostile response is predictive of poor outcome (Henry et al. 1986, 1990).

Handling Devaluation

Being devalued by a patient can be painful and is a frequent experience of therapists working with patients who have borderline or narcissistic psychopathology. The adaptive response of the therapist is to try to get the patient to understand the therapist's response as helpful and consistent with the goals of treatment rather than as retaliatory or as a way for the therapist to remove himself or herself as the object of the patient's aggression (Robbins 2000). The therapist must bind the affects and be aware of the countertransference responses elicited with the attack, including anger over the patient's display of narcissism.

> Patient: I needed that note from you, and you screwed up! I left word on your voice mail that I needed it by Monday [*vindictive tone*]. Figures, you could only get into medical school at a state school....
>
> Therapist 1 [*feels guilty*]: I'm really sorry. Next time I'll try to be more sensitive to your needs, but I was out on Monday. (*Masochistic countertransference response to what was actually an unreasonable demand, a mea culpa gratifying the patient's grandiose self*)
>
> Therapist 2 [*feels irritated*]: You're pretty quick to blame me and make critical comments, but you take no responsibility at all for what happened. You left the request over the weekend, and I was out on Monday. (*Accurate but critical rebuttal, which may leave the patient feeling demeaned and angry*)
>
> Patient: I've heard those excuses before! I needed you. Now, how can I trust you? I knew I should have gone to that Park Avenue shrink my mother told me about! He went to Harvard. He's quoted in the newspaper all the time.
>
> Therapist 3: Sometimes I'm going to disappoint you. It happens, even in the best relationships. It might scare you or make you angry that I'm not perfectly attuned to your needs, but fortunately, I don't need to be perfect to be helpful to you. I'll bet that other psychiatrist doesn't need to be perfect either to be effective. (*Authentic but measured response. Models healthy, adult behavior that is neither retaliating nor capitulating; clarifies the role of a "good-enough" therapist*)

The therapist must have appropriate training and the ability to understand feelings of irritation, frustration, and helplessness generated in response to a patient's chronic criticism and devaluation. Without adequate peer support or professional supervision, the therapist may become clinically disenchanted or disempowered and become either bored or overly confrontational (Rosenthal 2002).

Distancing from empathic connection is a common therapist response to patients' projective identifications (Kaufman 1992). Rather than identifying with the patient's projections and either capitulating or counterattacking, the therapist manages vulnerability and aggression in the context of being devalued. Such management is in concordance with supportive principles (Robbins 2000) and can allow the patient to establish an idealizing transference. The idealizing transference can enable the patient to experience safety in the relationship with the idealized therapist, which can serve as a corrective emotional experience (Alexander and French 1946). However, certain types of patients, such as help-rejecting complainers (see Chapter 5, "General Framework of Supportive Psychotherapy"), will maintain a transference position that is impermeable to therapist intervention and disclosure. Moreover, their pathogenic beliefs regarding self and others are confirmed by the therapist's repeated attempts to engage and problem solve (Sampson and Weiss 1986).

Conclusion

A robust therapeutic alliance is a strong predicator of positive outcome in psychotherapy—and in supportive psychotherapy, the alliance is posited as the foundation for therapeutic change; therefore, the clinician takes pains to promote and maintain the therapeutic alliance. In supportive psychotherapy, as in expressive psychotherapy, the clinician observes and tracks transference phenomena, but these phenomena are generally not a topic of discussion or interpretation in supportive psychotherapy unless the impact of negative transference is likely to interrupt treatment. The therapist typically uses clarification and confrontation in supportive treatment, but when interpretations are made, they tend to be incomplete or inexact. Because defenses are not confronted in supportive psychotherapy unless maladaptive, the clinician can learn to manage resistance with supportive techniques—and must always be alert to the potential role of countertransference so that it is properly managed and results in a better outcome.

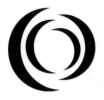

7

Crisis Intervention

History and Theory

Crisis intervention began during World War II out of a necessity to treat soldiers exposed to battlefield conditions. In World War I, soldiers with combat fatigue or shell shock (now called traumatic stress disorder) were quickly evacuated from the front lines, without treatment, despite observations that early intervention might reduce psychiatric morbidity (Salmon 1919). These soldiers often regressed or even became chronically impaired. In World War II, soldiers were treated at or near the front lines with crisis intervention techniques and were quickly returned to their combat units (Glass 1954).

During the time of World War II, Lindemann began working with survivors and relatives of survivors of the Cocoanut Grove nightclub fire in Boston; these individuals were experiencing acute grief and were unable to cope with their bereavement. In his seminal article, Lindemann (1944) described and contrasted normal and morbid grief. The survivors and their families were helped to do the necessary "grief work," which involved going through the mourning process and experiencing the loss. One of Lindemann's colleagues, Gerald Caplan (1961), began to work in the field of preventive psychiatry and helped develop the theoretical basis for the community mental health movement. Lindemann and Caplan were among the most important early theoreticians of the crisis intervention approach.

Parad and Parad (1990) defined *crisis* as an "upset in a steady state, a turning point leading to better or worse, a disruption or breakdown in a person's or family's normal or usual pattern of functioning" (pp. 3–4). A crisis occurs when an individual encounters a situation that leads to a breakdown in his or her usual pattern of functioning, creating disequilibrium. Generally, a crisis is precipitated by a hazardous event or a stressor, such as a catastrophe or disaster (e.g., earthquake, fire, war, terrorism), a relationship rupture or loss, rape, or abuse. A crisis may also result from a series of difficult events or mishaps rather than from one major occurrence, and a crisis can be a response to external and internal stress. During crises, individuals perceive their lives, needs, security, relationships, and sense of well-being to be at risk. Crises tend to be time limited, generally lasting no more than a few months; the duration depends on the stressor and on the individual's perception of and response to the stressor.

Crisis states can lead to personal growth rather than physical and psychological deterioration (Caplan 1961). Crisis makes growth possible because it assaults the individual's psychic structure and defenses, throwing them into a state of flux, which can make the individual more open to treatment. Davanloo (1980) incorporated production of a crisis into his short-term dynamic psychotherapy approach, viewing crisis as a means of disrupting ingrained defenses in order for patients to gain access to their inner lives and thereby change maladaptive ways of feeling, thinking, and behaving.

Crisis intervention is a therapeutic process aimed at restoring homeostatic balance and diminishing vulnerability to the stressor. Homeostasis is accomplished by the therapist's helping to mobilize the individual's abilities and social network and to promote adaptive coping mechanisms to reestablish equilibrium. Crisis intervention is a short-term approach that focuses on solving the immediate problem and includes the entire therapeutic repertoire for helping patients deal with the challenges and threats of overwhelming stress.

An individual's reaction to stress is the result of a number of factors, including age, health, personality issues, prior experience with stressful events, support and belief systems, and underlying biological or genetic vulnerability. Traumatic events are common and varied and can be personal, such as the death of a loved one, rape, the experience of being robbed, or involvement in a traffic accident. Other types of trauma, such as natural disasters or terrorist attacks, may involve large numbers of individuals, including persons not on the scene. In addition, the intensity and type of traumatic event are also important, as is an individual's coping ability. At times, a series of traumatic events may produce a crisis that a single event would not have provoked. For example, a series of losses might result in a crisis that did not occur after the first few losses. Losses include death, separation, illness, financial loss, and loss of employment, function, or status.

The distinction between crisis intervention and psychotherapy is often blurred, because the approaches may overlap in technique and length of treatment. Crisis intervention is generally expected to involve one to three contacts, whereas the duration of brief psychotherapy can extend from a few visits to 20 or more sessions. In this chapter, the term *crisis intervention* is also used for crisis-related treatment lasting longer than just a few sessions. This more inclusive form of crisis therapy is based on a number of different treatments, including dynamic supportive, cognitive-behavioral, humanistic, family, and systems approaches, as well as the use of medication when indicated. Systems approaches can be broad and can encompass actions such as working with and referral to social service agencies, clergy, mobile crisis units, suicide hotlines, and law enforcement agencies. In recent years, the focus of crisis intervention has been on emergency management and prevention through the use of various forms of debriefing.

Evaluation

According to Caplan (1961), ego assessment is key in the evaluation of an individual in a crisis situation. The evaluation consists of 1) examining the individual's capacity to deal with stress, maintain ego structure and equilibrium, and deal with reality; and 2) assessing problem-solving and coping abilities.

The evaluation of an individual in a crisis situation should be thorough and systematic but should also be essentially completed within the first session. A timely evaluation is critical; it enables the therapist to develop a case formulation and treatment plan and initiate treatment immediately. Indeed, even the evaluation session should be therapeutic, because the patient is in crisis and is seeking relief from suffering. The evaluation should follow the process outlined in Chapter 3, "Assessment, Case Formulation, and Goal Setting," but also should focus on the traumatic situation, precipitating event, and possible danger to self and others. The individual's experience of the trauma, including perceptions and feelings, is important, as is whether the person was a victim or a witness of the traumatic event. Also, the therapist should assess 1) the individual's current affect, anxiety level, and sense of hopefulness; and 2) the way in which he or she attempts to deal with the trauma.

The following vignette illustrates the evaluation process in a broad-based, supportive psychotherapy–crisis intervention approach (see Vignette 5, Session 1, on the DVD). The vignette includes excerpts from four sessions that began 6 months following the 2001 World Trade Center attack.

▶ Vignette 5: Crisis Intervention

▶ Session 1

William is a 44-year-old police officer with anxiety, depressive feelings, an inability to work, and difficulty enjoying anything about his life. He is tall, muscular, and physically imposing. In his first session, William reveals that he recently had a traumatic experience.

Therapist: So what's been troubling you?

William: I've just been having all kinds of problems in my life. I can't work...I can't sleep...I just don't enjoy anything anymore. (*Responds with multiple complaints*)

Therapist: So you're having trouble working and sleeping, and you're not finding any enjoyment in your life. How long have you been having these difficulties? (*Summarizes and attempts to find out when William's difficulties began*)

William: It's been going on for about 6 months, but it's gotten worse over the last couple of months, I'd say.

Therapist: I see that your problems began 6 months ago. What was happening at that time? (*Begins to focus on the beginning of the episode of illness*)

William: Nine-eleven happened. I was sent down there right at the beginning with three other policemen. It was terrible. I still can't believe what happened (*Begins to talk about the traumatic events that occurred on September 11, 2001*)

Therapist: Well, you know it is important that we try to go into as much detail as we can. I know it might be difficult for you, but can you tell me what happened when you were at the World Trade Center? (*Attempts to get details of the traumatic event and its effect on William*)

William: We got down there.... I was told to wait outside, and the other guys went in. They never came out.... I should have been there with them *[begins to cry]*! (*Is filled with emotion and perhaps feelings of guilt*)

Therapist: I can see that this is very difficult for you. (*Responds in an empathic manner*)

William: Yeah. I was told to stay outside and monitor traffic, to make sure that no civilians got into the buildings.

Therapist: You were outside, and they went in...and then what happened?

William: Well, I was standing there just looking up...I was stunned... I saw people jumping.

> ▶ **Vignette 5: Crisis Intervention** *(continued)*

Therapist: Oh my God! That must have been so frightening. *(Responds with emotion and in an empathic manner)*

William: Yeah.... I saw a man and a woman.... They were holding hands.... They were jumping *[begins to sob]*. *(Gives further information)*

Therapist: I'm so sorry.... You went through such a terrible ordeal. What a horror! I'm very sorry. *(Responds with emotion and in an empathic manner)*

William: That was only the first part of it. Then all of a sudden, the buildings began to shake and then—I couldn't believe it—they started to come down, and I was buried! And all of a sudden, I looked up, and I saw my wife and my son holding hands and smiling and waving at me.... I thought I was dead.

Therapist: So you were buried, and you saw your wife and your son. You thought you were dead. How did you get through that experience? *(Responds with a clarification, tracking, and admiration, and continues exploring)*

William: At first I was completely paralyzed.... I couldn't reason. My mind was totally confused.... I felt like a mummy.... I didn't move right away.

Therapist: And then what happened?

William: I reached for my eyes, and I started to pull the stuff out of my eyes and ears, and I stood up and I realized I was actually alive. I don't know how I got out.... I saw a woman. She was on her knees, and she had blood coming out of her forehead. I picked her up, and I took her to a rescue area. Then I went back in and found another man, and I carried him out also. *(Despite his horrendous ordeal, William behaved in a heroic manner.)*

Therapist: So you helped rescue two people! After everything you'd gone through, you rescued two people! *(Praises and expresses admiration for his heroic behavior)*

William: Yes, but I...the guys I came with...they never got out. I should have been there with them. I keep thinking about it. *(Despite his heroic behavior and the therapist's praise and admiration, William indicates that he feels guilty about not going in with the other policemen.)*

Therapist: You were a hero—and yet you still believe that you should have been with them. Losing three fellow officers must have been very devastating for you. *(Praises and begins to address the issue of William surviving while his fellow officers all died)*

> **Vignette 5: Crisis Intervention** *(continued)*

This vignette illustrates part of the process of evaluating a patient who is in a crisis situation and has a traumatic stress disorder. In the remainder of the evaluation, the therapist explores William's guilt about staying behind while others went in, his level of anxiety, and the extent of his depression. William's current family situation is examined, as well as his history. The following information emerges.

> The patient has been extremely anxious and tearful following his traumatic experience. He has been pacing back and forth in his home and thinking constantly about what happened to him on September 11, 2001. He has startle reactions to loud noises and has flashbacks about the building collapsing, people jumping, and seeing his wife and son. William has nightmares and so avoids sleep. He can no longer concentrate, has little energy, feels helpless, and no longer enjoys anything in his life. He has been unable to return to work and tries to avoid anything that might remind him of September 11. His previous performance at work was quite good, and he was decorated on several occasions for heroism.
>
> William grew up in a middle-class family and had a good relationship with his mother. When he was 15 years old, his father died. William's relationship with his father had been difficult and filled with conflict, which resulted in mixed feelings toward his father. These feelings did not resolve when his father was dying, and they may have played a role in William's emphasis on bodybuilding and on presenting a strong manly image.

The therapist concludes that William has posttraumatic stress disorder (PTSD). Before the trauma, the patient was functioning at a high level and had good coping skills despite unresolved problems with his father. At present, his coping skills are no longer adequate, but he has a supportive spouse and appears to be motivated for psychotherapy. The treatment goals, formulated with the patient, include amelioration of his symptoms and a return to work. The treatment plan includes development of a supportive, positive therapeutic relationship at the onset of treatment, followed by work on symptom reduction with the use of exposure therapy, along with cognitive restructuring. Medication for anxiety and depression, such as a selective serotonin reuptake inhibitor, may also be indicated. As treatment progresses, a major focus will be to help him return to work as soon as possible.

Treatment

The therapeutic approaches used in crisis intervention are primarily those of brief supportive psychotherapy, consisting of maintenance of focus and a high therapist activity level; use of clearly established goals, a time limit, and a number of supportive and cognitive-behavioral interventions; and most important, establishment of a solid therapeutic alliance. A number of systematic approaches to crisis intervention have been described (James and Gilliland 2001; Puryear 1979; Roberts 2000).

Systematic approaches to crisis intervention all stress assessment, patient safety, establishment of rapport and hopefulness, supportive interventions, and positive actions and plans. The importance of assessment was discussed in the previous section, "Evaluation." Patient safety is part of the assessment process and should be monitored throughout therapy if the individual's safety is in question (see the section "Suicide" later in this chapter). Establishing rapport and promoting hopefulness are important in all forms of psychotherapy and are major factors in fostering the therapeutic alliance. The therapeutic alliance has been shown to be the best predictor of success in psychotherapy (Gaston 1990; Horvath and Symonds 1991). The major elements of the alliance (Gaston 1990) are the patient's affective bond with the therapist, the patient's ability to work purposefully and collaboratively with the therapist, the therapist's empathic understanding and involvement, and the agreement of patient and therapist on the goals and tasks of therapy. The use of supportive or empathic interventions helps promote the alliance, making it possible to use exposure techniques to help resolve the patient's reaction to the trauma. Positive actions and plans provide the patient with structure and improve self-esteem and hope for the future. Vignette 5 on the DVD continues, including Sessions 2, 4, and 5 with William, the police officer with PTSD resulting from the events of September 11, 2001. These sessions illustrate the treatment process in a broad-based supportive psychotherapy crisis intervention approach.

▶ Vignette 5: Crisis Intervention *(continued)*

▶ Session 2

William has completed his first session of supportive psychotherapy crisis intervention. In addition, treatment with a selective serotonin reuptake inhibitor has been started, with the dose gradually being increased to a therapeutic level during the course of treatment. The next two sessions are primarily directed at forming a secure and positive therapeutic alliance through the use of supportive interventions. Part of the patient's second session follows.

▶ Vignette 5: Crisis Intervention *(continued)*

William: My wife told me that I don't bother with her anymore, that I just ignore her—but I don't feel like talking about anything, doing anything.... I just don't feel like talking. *(Begins with a complaint from his wife rather than continuing to discuss the traumatic event; possibly a defensive move)*

Therapist: You know last week at our first meeting, we explored what happened to you on that terrible day of 9/11, and something about your past life, and a bit concerning your relationship with your wife and son, and maybe today we can go into your current relationship with Cathy more in-depth. *(Chooses to address William's current issue with his wife to build a therapeutic relationship before going back to the traumatic event, which William may not be ready for at the current time)*

William: Well...Cathy comes over to me and tries to talk to me...to get me started talking, but I don't feel like talking; it's still too difficult. *(Indicates that he is overwhelmed, which may have implications for his feelings about talking to the therapist)*

Therapist: So it's really hard for you to talk, and I understand this. Perhaps there are some things that would be easier for you to talk about. *(Responds in an empathic manner and asks William to focus on areas that are less painful, anxiety provoking, and conflictual)*

William: It is really hard to talk about 9/11...I like to talk about my son...I guess some things around the house. I like to do some gardening.

Therapist: So you could talk to Cathy about those things—about the house, your son, and so forth. Can you give me an example of what you might feel comfortable talking with Cathy about?

The therapist has recognized that the patient is having difficulty talking at home and is possibly having difficulty talking with the therapist. However, because the patient is talking spontaneously, the therapist has decided not to address the therapeutic relationship and instead has begun to focus on concrete areas that the patient can discuss with his wife. Focusing on concrete areas helps to reduce anxiety, which is important in both supportive psychotherapy and crisis intervention.

William: Cathy wants Billy to go to sleep-away camp. I don't know—he's not much of an athlete, but he does like to play the saxophone. I kind of think it would be better if he just stayed home. *(Indicates his wish to have Billy at home with him)*

Therapist: Could it be that you disagree with Cathy because you would really like Billy to stay home with you? *(Clarification, expressed tentatively)*

> ### ▶ **Vignette 5: Crisis Intervention** *(continued)*

William: I do like having him around. *(Ignores his conflict with Cathy and focuses on Billy)*

Therapist: Yeah. So maybe I would be correct in saying that you want Billy to be with you, but you find it hard to speak to Cathy about this directly? *(Brings William back to his conflict with Cathy; using a supportive approach, asks if he agrees)*

William: That makes sense. I just can't be clear about what it is that I want, because I just really don't know. *(Agrees but indicates that he becomes passive and indecisive with Cathy)*

Therapist: It sounds like you would like to have Billy home this summer, but it's hard for you to be direct with Cathy, so you hang back and yet get annoyed with her. Is this correct? Do you agree with that? *(Interprets William's wish to have Billy home and William's defensive posture of passivity and distraction accompanied by annoyance with Cathy; again employs the supportive technique of asking for feedback so that William is not overwhelmed)*

The therapist has asked for a specific example of William's difficulty in communicating with his wife. Obtaining specific concrete examples from patients is always preferable to leaving things on a general level. When patients generalize, it is difficult to understand what they have in mind. In addition, it is not helpful to patients to remain in a confused or unclear state.

Having understood that William wishes to have his son at home, the therapist has been able to clarify this wish with William. The therapist has used a number of supportive approaches. Instead of addressing the transference, the therapist has continued to concentrate on the patient's current life and his difficulty with his wife, Cathy. In supportive psychotherapy, the transference generally is not addressed unless it is negative. Instead, the therapist concentrates on current issues in the patient's life and on the real relationship with the therapist. Clarification is used as a supportive technique because it does not place demands or therapist expectations on the patient. In addition, the therapist has been able to link William's avoidance and annoyance with his wife to his wish to keep Billy home for the summer and not have him go off to camp as his wife wishes.

The pursuit of affect is generally avoided in supportive psychotherapy and has been avoided in this session. However, William's emotional experiences resulting from the World Trade Center tragedy will need to be addressed when exposure techniques are used later in therapy.

▶ **Vignette 5: Crisis Intervention** *(continued)*

The therapist has determined that a good therapeutic relationship was established during the first three sessions (Session 3 is not shown on the DVD). Therefore, exposure therapy within a supportive framework can now be attempted to enable the patient to work through his traumatic experience, as shown in the following Sessions 4 and 5.

▶ **Session 4**

Therapist: William, I thought that we might go back and explore what happened to you on 9/11. If we can look at your experience together, it should help you to better deal with it and move on with your life. How do you feel about doing that now? *(Asks for William's agreement to explore his traumatic experience. Asking for agreement constitutes the supportive technique of agenda setting.)*

William: If it can help. I think I'm more ready.

Therapist: It's good that you feel ready and that we're able to proceed. Let's go back to that day when you went to the World Trade Center. OK? *(Praises William and continues to involve him as a partner in planning the discussion)*

William: OK.

Therapist: You and your fellow officers were sent to the World Trade Center about when? *(Begins a detailed exploration of William's traumatic experience)*

William: In the morning, after the second plane hit…we drove up.

Therapist: And as you were driving up, what were you experiencing?

William: The fires were just raging…. We knew by then that it was an attack. We met the sergeant, and he told me I should stay outside to keep people out…as I said before.

Therapist: What was it like for you, remaining outside while the others went in? *(Is aware of William's not wanting to remain behind and his guilt feelings about being the only survivor from his group)*

William: I wanted to go in with them.

Therapist: So how did you feel? *(For the first time the therapist asks about William's feelings. Exposure therapy relies on the patient's experiencing and exploring feelings, in a somewhat controlled fashion, during the session.)*

William: Standing around I felt useless…. I was annoyed. I didn't want to stay behind.

Therapist: That's understandable, but you were ordered to stay behind. *(Absolution as a supportive technique)*

> ▶ **Vignette 5: Crisis Intervention** *(continued)*

The therapist has emphasized that William was ordered to stay behind because during the evaluation session William indicated that he felt guilty and conflicted about staying outside. The therapist is preparing the groundwork for addressing William's cognitive distortion of this issue and his possible survivor guilt.

The session continues with a recounting of the traumatic events that followed.

> William: I was standing there...in the street. Then all of a sudden, I saw people jumping from the building. Some of them were on fire.
>
> Therapist: That's horrible! What were you feeling? *(Asks William for his feelings in an empathic manner to promote exploration and desensitization)*
>
> William: It was hard to look.... *[begins to sob]* I couldn't believe it. Then I saw a man and a woman jumping.... They were holding hands *[becomes visibly shaken and anxious]*!
>
> Therapist: Who wouldn't be devastated, shaken, and tearful? *(Clarifies in an empathic manner using the supportive technique of normalizing)*

The therapist has been obtaining a detailed account of William's traumatic experience and has also been monitoring the patient's level of anxiety so that the anxiety will remain within manageable limits. If a patient's anxiety level gets too high, the therapist can slow down the account and initiate anxiety-lowering interventions, such as having the patient engage in progressive muscular relaxation and deep breathing. In addition to these techniques, which are generally used in exposure therapy, supportive interventions such as reassurance can be used.

The session continued with a detailed exploration of the patient's experiences of that day, including the collapse of the buildings, his near burial in the debris, his hallucination of his wife and son, and his belief that he was dead. The therapist elicits these experiences in great detail and in an empathic manner, with careful monitoring of the patient's anxiety level. During the exploration of William's vision of his wife and son—the vision in which he saw them holding hands and waving good-bye to him—William becomes visibly shaken and anxious because at that time he believed he was dead. The therapist stops the exploration and begins anxiety-lowering techniques such as deep breathing.

> ▶ **Vignette 5: Crisis Intervention** *(continued)*

▶ **Session 5**

Session 5 begins with a discussion of the patient's anxiety level during the interval between sessions. This information is important because the aim in supportive therapy is to keep anxiety level as low as possible. William indicates that he has not been experiencing a significant amount of anxiety between sessions.

> Therapist: Do you think you feel ready now to continue exploring what happened to you on that day on 9/11? *(Checks to see if William is ready to continue exposure therapy; again uses the supportive technique of agenda setting)*
> William: Yeah…I can keep going.
> Therapist: You're very strong, and you have a lot of resilience. So, let's pick up where we left off: after you saw your wife and son. Is that OK? *(Offers praise—a supportive intervention—and then resumes exploration of William's traumatic experience)*
> William: Yeah, I began to realize that I wasn't actually dead, and I started to push away all the stuff off me…out of my face, ears, and eyes. It was all over me. *(Continues without much difficulty)*
> Therapist: So as you began to realize you were not dead, how did you feel?
> William: I certainly felt some relief.… I thought, thank God—thank God, I'm all right. Then I got up and I saw a woman on her knees. She was bleeding from her scalp, blood was coming down her face. All I thought to do was help her up and carry her out to the rescue area.
> Therapist: Yeah. So despite your being battered and even thinking you were dead just a few minutes earlier, you were still able to pull a woman out of the rubble and rescue her. That's amazing! *(Offers praise and expresses admiration—both useful supportive interventions, provided the praise and admiration are clearly reality based and deserved)*

The therapist goes on to explore the details of the patient's next few hours after he picked himself up from the rubble. These details include rescuing a man, going to the hospital to have lacerations sutured, and finding out that the three policemen who went into the building died. All these experiences are fully explored during the next few sessions, until William can talk about his experience without too much anxiety or overwhelming sadness.

> ### ▶ Vignette 5: Crisis Intervention *(continued)*

William's treatment involves the use of exposure therapy in the context of a supportive relationship. The therapist is able to take the patient through his traumatic experience in a slow and detailed manner over the course of several meetings. The therapist monitors William's anxiety level so that he is not overwhelmed. If the patient begins to become overly aroused, the therapist stops the exposure work and uses a number of supportive techniques, such as praise, reassurance, and relaxation therapy. At the same time, a great deal of work is required to restructure William's excessive feelings of guilt about being the only survivor of his group of four policemen. The therapist challenges William's self-blaming cognitions to help him reframe his idea that he should have been inside the World Trade Center with his fellow officers. The therapist helps William understand the concept of survivor guilt when she states, "Many people who survive tragedies as you did feel guilty."

After 10 sessions, William gradually improves and is able to return to work and to feel comfortable with his wife and son. He still has episodes of anxiety and sadness, which he is able to manage, and he continues taking medication. He has two follow-up sessions, 1 month later and then 3 months later, to prevent relapse.

Suicide

The prediction of suicide is problematic because there is no reliable way of determining suicidal risk in a given individual (Fawcett et al. 1993; Pokorny 1983). Two major problems occur when attempts are made to predict suicide: identification of too many false-positive cases, and oversight of many instances of completed suicide. Nevertheless, more than 90% of completed suicides occur in individuals with a recent major psychiatric illness (Fawcett et al. 1993). The most common diagnoses are major depression, chronic alcoholism and drug abuse, schizophrenia, borderline personality disorder, bipolar disorder, and eating disorders. A careful and thorough assessment of the suicidal patient is critical to determine the diagnosis and the proper treatment approach. Crisis intervention approaches, generally accompanied by the use of medication, often play an important role in the treatment of suicidal individuals.

Assessment of Risk

Suicidal thoughts and behaviors are so common that it is essential to ask all patients about suicidal ideas and attempts. A history of suicide attempts increases a person's risk for suicide. Individuals who have well-defined plans to kill themselves are at greater risk than individuals with vague or poorly formulated plans. When a suicidal person has the means to end his or her life (e.g., owns a firearm), the patient is at significant risk. The presence of strong family support or a significant other can have a mitigating effect on suicidal risk. Hopelessness, pessimism, aggression, impulsiveness, and psychic anxiety are poor prognostic signs. Another factor to be considered is the loss of a significant other through separation, divorce, or death.

Paradoxically, it was found that more than half of patients who died by suicide had consulted clinicians within 1 year before death and had denied suicidal thoughts or indicated that they rarely occurred (Clark and Fawcett 1992). Often, these same patients communicated directly or indirectly to a close friend or relative that they were thinking of ending their lives. This information suggests that physicians should routinely question close relatives and friends of patients who may be at risk for suicide.

Fawcett et al. (1990, 1993) divided suicidal risk into acute and chronic categories. Individuals who are at acute risk often have severe anxiety, thoughts about negative events occurring, insomnia, anhedonia, agitation, and alcohol abuse (Busch et al. 2003). Persons at more chronic risk have more-typical risk factors, such as suicidal ideation and plans, and a history of suicide attempts.

The risk of suicide is often greatest during the week after hospital admission and the month after discharge and during the early period of recovery from a psychiatric disorder (Hawton 1987).

Treatment

Once an individual has been determined to be acutely suicidal, hospitalization may be indicated. If hospitalization is not feasible or not absolutely necessary, the therapist should enlist the aid of significant others who can spend time with the patient and not leave the patient alone. The therapist needs to be available for contact either by the patient or by the patient's family or friends, and should provide them with information regarding 24-hour hotlines and the nearest emergency room. Medication is often necessary to relieve the patient's anxiety, agitation, or depression. The frequency of treatment sessions will vary, depending on the patient's needs. Some patients may need to be seen daily for ongoing support and structure. Accordingly, it is important that the same clinician see the patient throughout the period of crisis intervention. Important issues on which to focus are patient hopelessness and pessimism. Supportive approaches involving praise, reassurance, and cognitive restructuring are often useful to help enhance self-esteem by counteracting negative or distorted cognitions about the self. As always, establishment and maintenance of a positive therapeutic alliance are essential.

Crisis Intervention Versus Psychotherapy

As stated in the section "History and Theory" at the beginning of this chapter, crisis intervention theory is based on a number of psychological approaches, including dynamic supportive psychotherapy, cognitive-behavioral therapy, humanistic treatments, family therapy, and systems approaches. Crisis intervention is time limited and is not focused on psychological insight, personality issues, or psychiatric disorders. An individual receiving crisis intervention is generally in transition or has lost his or her equilibrium because of a traumatic experience that has disrupted his or her life. The objective is to help the individual deal with the stressful period, achieve stability, and return to his or her precrisis level of functioning, or if the patient needs further treatment, move on to the next level of care.

Crisis intervention differs from psychotherapy in a number of ways (outlined in Table 7–1). Crisis treatment is given as soon as possible and in close proximity to the stressor or traumatic event. It is time limited, and the therapist is active, supportive, and directive. As in supportive psychotherapy (as opposed to expressive psychotherapy), the focus is on the here and now rather than on the past or on transference issues.

Critical Incident Stress Management

Critical incident stress management (CISM) was originally developed for use with emergency workers; however, its scope has been expanded to include anyone exposed to severe trauma (Everly and Mitchell 1999; Mitchell and Everly 2003). CISM is a comprehensive and integrated crisis intervention approach for individuals and groups. The components of CISM are summarized in Table 7–2 and include the following: precrisis preparation involving stress management education and training for individuals and groups of professional and emergency workers; briefings on disasters and terrorist or other large-scale incidents for rescue workers and civilians; defusing (i.e., immediate small-group discussion) to ensure assessment and triage and to mitigate symptoms; critical incident stress debriefing (CISD) (Mitchell and Everly 1996) to reduce impairments from traumatic stress, facilitate closure, and mitigate symptoms for individuals and groups; individual or family crisis intervention; and follow-up and referral for further assessment and treatment.

Table 7–1. Crisis intervention versus psychotherapy

	Crisis intervention	Psychotherapy
Context	Prevention	Reparation
Timing	Immediate; close temporal relationship to stressor or acute decompensation	Delayed; distant from stressor or acute decompensation
Location	Close proximity to stressor or acute decompensation; anywhere needed	Safe, secure environment
Duration	Typically one to three contacts	As long as needed or desired
Provider's role	Active, directive	Guiding, collaborative, consultative
Strategic foci	Conscious processes, environmental stressors or factors	Conscious and unconscious sources of pathogenesis
Temporal focus	Here and now	Present and past
Patient expectations	Symptom reduction, reduction of impairment, directive support	Symptom reduction, reduction of impairment, personal growth, guidance, collaboration
Goals	Stabilization, reduction of impairment, a return to function or a shift to next level of care	Symptom reduction, reduction of impairment, correction of pathogenesis, personal growth, personal reconstruction

Source. Aguilera et al. 1970; Artiss 1963; Everly and Mitchell 1998; Koss and Shiang 1994; Salmon 1919; Sandoval 1985; Skaikeu 1990; Spiegel and Classen 1995; Wilkinson and Vera 1985.
Reprinted from Everly GS Jr, Mitchell JT: *Critical Incident Stress Management (CISM): A New Era and Standard of Care in Crisis Intervention,* 2nd Edition. Ellicott City, MD, Chevron Publishing, 1999. Used with permission.

Table 7–2. Core components of critical incident stress management

Intervention	Timing	Activation	Goals	Recipients
Precrisis preparation	Precrisis	Driven by crisis anticipation	Setting of expectations, improved coping, stress management	Individuals, groups, organizations
Demobilization and staff consultation (rescuers)	Shift disengagement	Event driven	Presentation of information, consultation, psychological decompression, stress management	Organizations, large groups
Crisis management briefing (civilians, schools, businesses)	Anytime postcrisis	Event driven	Presentation of information, consultation, psychological decompression, stress management	Organizations, large groups
Defusing	Postcrisis (within 12 hours)	Usually symptom driven	Symptom mitigation, possible closure, triage	Small groups
Critical incident stress debriefing	Postcrisis (1–10 days; mass disasters: 3–4 weeks)	Usually symptom driven; sometimes event driven	Facilitation of psychological closure, symptom mitigation, triage	Individuals, small groups
Individual crisis intervention	Anytime, anywhere	Symptom driven	Symptom mitigation, possible return to function, referral if needed	Individuals
Family crisis intervention	Anytime	Symptom or event driven	Fostering of support and communication	Families

Table 7-2. Core components of critical incident stress management (*continued*)

Intervention	Timing	Activation	Goals	Recipients
Community and organizational consultation	Anytime	Symptom or event driven	Symptom mitigation, possible closure, referral if needed	Organizations
Pastoral crisis intervention	Anytime	Usually symptom driven	"Crisis of faith" mitigation, use of spiritual tools to assist in recovery	Individuals, families, groups
Follow-up and referral	Anytime	Usually symptom driven	Mental status assessment, a shift to higher level of care if needed	Individuals, families

Source. Adapted from Everly GS Jr, Mitchell JT: *Critical Incident Stress Management (CISM): A New Era and Standard of Care in Crisis Intervention,* 2nd Edition. Ellicott City, MD, Chevron Publishing, 1999. Used with permission.

A typical CISD approach after a traumatic event involves a group of victims who undergo the interventions, listed above, in a single 1- to 3-hour session. The efficacy of a single-session debriefing in preventing PTSD or other disorders has recently come into question. In a meta-analysis of single-session debriefing within 1 month after trauma, van Emmerik et al. (2002) found that CISD interventions do not improve natural recovery from psychological trauma. However, single-session approaches of this sort may help reduce immediate distress and facilitate referral of patients for further treatment. Positive outcomes have been achieved with cognitive-behavioral treatments that were administered within the first month of the traumatic incident and that involved education, exposure, and cognitive restructuring (Bryant et al. 1999; Foa 1997; Foa et al. 1991).

Conclusion

In this chapter, we provided a brief history and the theoretical background of crisis intervention. Individuals exposed to severe trauma can react in a number of ways, and some of these reactions necessitate crisis intervention. A thorough evaluation of a patient presenting in crisis is always necessary. Treatment approaches vary depending on the needs of the patient, but generally include supportive interventions, exposure therapy, and cognitive restructuring. Therapists must pay particular attention to establishing and maintaining a positive therapeutic alliance. The terrorist attacks of September 11, 2001, in New York and Washington, D.C.; the 2010 Haiti earthquake; and in 2011, the shooting of Rep. Gabrielle Giffords, the Japan earthquake and tsunami, and the severe tornadoes and floods in the Midwest have made both the general public and mental health professionals more aware of these issues and the need for crisis intervention services.

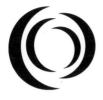

8

Applicability to
Special Populations

Severe Mental Illness

As originally conceived, supportive psychotherapy was indicated for patients with severe mental illness, as well as for other patients for whom expressive treatment was not indicated. The original indication for supportive psychotherapy was treatment at the extreme supportive end of the supportive-expressive psychotherapy continuum described in Chapter 1, "The Concept of Supportive Psychotherapy." This form of supportive treatment was focused primarily on improving deficient ego functions, reducing anxiety, and preventing downward social drift due to loss of adaptive skills and increasing isolation. In addition to offering the patient an understanding, supportive relationship, this approach contained many of the following techniques: advice, reassurance, exhortation, praise, encouragement, lending ego, and environmental manipulation. Shoring up of defenses was the default mode, confrontation was rare, and interpretation did not occur.

In current practice, even for patients who are quite impaired because of severe mental illness, therapists should strive for a balance between supportive and expressive elements in supportive treatment. Depending on several factors—including the degree of stabilization after acute exacerbation of illness, the strength of the therapeutic alliance (see Chapter 6, "The Therapeutic Relationship"), and the patient's treatment goals—confrontation and, at times, interpretation can be useful techniques in supportive psychotherapy. Cognitive learning strategies, such as teaching, using slogans, modeling, and giving anticipatory guidance, are commonly used. The treatment components of psychoeducation and skills training, which have been framed as independent interventions, are consistent with the model of supportive treatment and are particularly useful in supportive psychotherapy for chronic mental illness.

Schizophrenia

Schizophrenia is the prototypical severe mental illness. When treating a patient who has schizophrenia, the therapist provides education about the illness, promotes medication compliance, facilitates reality testing, encourages problem solving by the patient, and reinforces adaptive behavior with praise (Lamberti and Herz 1995). Gunderson et al. (1984) demonstrated that patients with schizophrenia have better treatment retention and better outcome when given weekly supportive treatment rather than more intensive expressive treatment.

Praise is a form of reinforcement that can support the patient's self-esteem and motivation for adaptive change. As described in detail in Chapter 4, "Techniques," praise is an important esteem-building technique. However, praise builds self-esteem only when the praised behavior is considered praiseworthy by the patient. Therefore, the therapist must understand what the patient will find worthy of praise. The therapist also must attempt to understand what the patient finds rewarding in addition to praise, so that these incentives can be enlisted to provide positive feedback. Determining what the patient finds rewarding is especially important at the left side of the psychopathology continuum (e.g., in schizophrenia), where positive reinforcement is an important factor in maintaining the therapeutic alliance and motivating engagement in treatment. Positive reinforcement is helpful for patients with schizophrenia because they commonly have neurocognitive impairments; negative symptoms, such as apathy, anhedonia, and poor motivation; and poor insight. A reinforcer can be a favorite food, activity, person, or social event that increases the strength or frequency of the patient's contingent behavior. Properly assessed and delivered reinforcers increase patients' skill acquisition, achievement of goals, and self-esteem (Lecomte et al. 2000). External rewards that patients value may be helpful in engaging and maintaining these patients in treatment. Rewards can include subway tokens, certificates of accomplishment, a celebratory event, and gift certificates. Administration of accurate praise, as described throughout this book, is an effective and inexpensive reward.

Psychoeducation

Typically, supportive psychotherapy for patients with severe mental illness includes psychoeducation about the illness, its trajectory, and its treatment. The literature suggests that educating patients about their schizophrenia or substance dependence reinforces psychosocial rehabilitation (Goldman and Quinn 1988). Most patients find learning new information generally to be supportive. When provided in an empathic way, psychoeducation offers the patient a new cognitive structure on which to base more-realistic decision making. Psychoeducation also gives the patient an explanation of or rationale for symptoms and suffering; giving such explanations or rationales may also bolster the patient's self-esteem.

In addition, concrete information about the illness arms the patient with practical knowledge that can help improve his or her ability to cope with chronic illness—an adaptive skill. For example, early in an exacerbation of the manic phase of bipolar disorder, the patient frequently loses the capacity to understand that his or her judgment is impaired by mania. During a remission, the psychiatrist can teach the patient that sleeping even 1 hour less than usual for 2 nights in a row may be an early sign of relapse into mania. This information gives the patient an opportunity to demonstrate some adaptive mastery over the illness and to act before an exacerbation can impair judgment and destroy the chance to "step on the brakes." For example, when the symptom of impaired sleep occurs and the patient contacts the psychiatrist for a dose escalation of antimanic medication, the patient will likely experience increased self-efficacy and self-esteem. These positive effects will occur as a result of the patient's sense of increased competence in anticipating potentially damaging future events and will strengthen the therapeutic alliance.

Supporting Adaptive Skills

To help patients who have impairments in interpersonal functioning secondary to severe mental disorders such as schizophrenia, the therapist can integrate behavioral skills training and other cognitive-behavioral techniques into supportive psychotherapy. The model of change in supportive therapy is change through learning and through introjection of or identification with an accepting, well-related therapist (Pinsker et al. 1991). Training in social and independent living skills for patients with severe mental illness is an approach grounded in learning principles, wherein the therapist breaks down complex social repertoires and models correct behavior for the patient, who repeatedly practices the skills after learning them. After the steps are assembled, the patient practices the complex interaction—first with the therapist, then in the real world. The therapist uses supportive techniques, such as behavioral-goal setting, encouragement, modeling, shaping, and praise (positive reinforcement), to teach interpersonal skills

(Glynn et al. 2002). This activity directly supports adaptive skills and builds patients' self-esteem. Studies have demonstrated the utility of these interventions in improving social competence (Heinssen et al. 2000; Lauriello et al. 1999).

Patients with schizophrenia have social skills deficits, which may be a result of impaired information processing. Skills training uses the problem-solving, repetitive, and practical approach of supportive psychotherapy and is effective in improving basic conversational skills, recreational skills, medication management, and management of symptoms (Liberman et al. 1998; Smith et al. 1999). A related cognitive-behavioral approach, relapse prevention, is discussed in the section "Adaptive Skills and Relapse Prevention" later in this chapter.

At times, the clinician must balance his or her focus on anxiety reduction as a major supportive strategy with the patient's determination to work through a particular problem, which could increase the patient's adaptive skills. For example, a patient might become anxious on hearing certain information about schizophrenia from the therapist. However, providing guidance about hearing the information and reframing the content in an attempt to shore up the patient's coping skills may reduce the patient's anxiety. Having more extensive coping strategies that use higher-level defenses (e.g., rationalization) can mean that the patient has a more flexible and adaptive approach to his or her illness. At other times, when the patient signals that he or she is experiencing too much anxiety to deal with a subject directly, it can be useful for the therapist to attempt to "back into" discussion of the difficult topic.

> Therapist: So, I would like to talk to you about what you understand about your illness. Is that OK with you? (*"Shows the map" before exploring the territory*)
>
> Patient: I guess.
>
> Therapist: If what I'm saying doesn't make sense to you, please tell me, and I'll try to clarify it. If it makes you more nervous, let me know, and we'll talk about something else. OK? (*Offers anticipatory guidance about material to be explored, gives patient permission to stop the exploration, sets a collaborative tone, and indicates that therapist is sensitive to patient's feelings*)
>
> Patient: All right.
>
> Therapist: Has anyone discussed with you what your diagnosis is? That means the medical name of the illness that's bringing you into psychiatric treatment.
>
> Patient: Uh, depression. I have depression.
>
> Therapist: That's what they told you?
>
> Patient: I don't know...um, I have depression. (*Patient has been told previously that his diagnosis is schizophrenia. He is either being evasive or using denial.*)

Therapist: Could you describe for me what the word *depression* means to you?

Patient: Yeah, I couldn't sleep, and I don't do much. Don't feel like it. I used to do things.

Therapist: Any other problems, like in your thoughts or feelings?

Patient: I have depression. *(Concrete, perseverative, nonelaborative answer)*

Therapist: Are you sad a lot? People who are depressed are often sad.

Patient: No, not sad. I just don't feel much of anything. Tired. I don't know. *(Disclaims a low mood associated with depression)*

Therapist: OK. Now, other than being tired, are there things you've been experiencing lately that have caused you problems?

Patient: Huh? Like what? *[suspicious look]*

Therapist: Well, you told the other doctor back in your intake evaluation that you had been thinking that somebody or maybe some group was trying to harm you, that you saw evidence of that. Is that accurate?

Patient: That was before. I don't think about it now. *[looks away] (Engages in distancing and avoiding)*

Therapist: Can you tell me a little about what you were thinking and experiencing then? *(Asks about patient's experience)*

Patient: Scary, uh...don't want to talk about it. I don't think about it now. *(Focusing on persecutory delusion increases patient's anxiety.)*

Therapist: OK, I won't ask you about the details. So, now it's not on your mind. You said it was before. Before when? I didn't understand what you meant. *(Moves away from past experience; asks for clarification of patient's statement)*

Patient: You know, when I went on the pills for depression, it got better.

Therapist: Ah, so you don't have those scary thoughts so much since you started taking the medication? It's good you're taking it! *(Clarifies, connecting medication and relief from delusional thinking; adds praise)*

Patient: Yeah. That's true.

Therapist: So, let me clarify: the medication you're taking seems to have a good impact on scary thoughts and experiences. Is that accurate?

Patient: That's true. *[eye contact, brightens a little]*

Therapist: So I guess it's a good idea to keep taking it? *(Ties what patient experiences as beneficial to a motivating statement for medication adherence)*

Patient: Yeah!...And I talk to people better. They don't seem so negative to me. *(Validates therapist's position)*

Therapist: So the medication helps you communicate better, too? Does that mean you get along with people better than before?

Patient: I keep to myself pretty much. But I don't get into fights like I did. *(Is more elaborative as anxiety is reduced in situ)*

Therapist: You mean you got into physical fights?

Patient: Only one time. Mostly just yelling back at some of the people when I knew what they were up to.

Therapist: What were they up to? *(Asks for clarification)*

Patient: They were trying to make me look bad—said bad things about me from down the street. *[looks away]* Hmm, I don't think about it now. **(Starts to demonstrate increased anxiety, repeating his reflexive phrase)**

Therapist: So that's better now, too? That's good. What else is better? **(Goes along with the resistance; moves back to the present to reduce anxiety)**

Patient: My walls are quiet. I sleep better.

Therapist: How were they noisy?

Patient: The lady upstairs was making noise at night.

Therapist: What kind of noises? Like playing music too loud? Moving furniture?

Patient: No, uh, she would say ugly, ugly things to me. I couldn't sleep; I'd have to stay up.

Therapist: How would she talk to you?

Patient: I don't know—but it came from the wall.

Therapist: So you were hearing her voice telling you things you found unpleasant and you couldn't sleep? And it's better now? **(Clarifies)**

Patient: Yes, I can sleep again.

Therapist: That must have been a terrible time for you. I'm glad you're feeling better. What a relief that must be! **(Gives an empathic response based on patient's statements)**

Patient: Uh-huh. *[smiles]*

Therapist: I'm going to summarize what you've told me the medication does for you, so we're clear I have it right. It takes away scary thoughts and experiences, takes away voices at night and helps you to sleep, and lets you get along with people better.

Patient: That's it.

Therapist: Sounds like good medicine!

Patient: It works.

Therapist: So can we get back to that illness that gave you the scary thoughts and experiences like voices, that kept you up, and that made it hard to get along with people? **(Again "shows the map")**

Patient: OK.

Therapist: The medicine you are taking treats those symptoms of a disorder called schizophrenia—and, as we've just talked about, treats them pretty well: you're feeling a lot better than before.

Patient: I don't have that! My face didn't change. I don't attack people and drink their blood. My face didn't change. **(Becomes anxious and derails; reveals his delusional fears)**

Therapist: I think maybe you're confusing an idea you have about vampires— that maybe you saw on TV—with schizophrenia. Vampires aren't real. Schizophrenia is, but it's a treatable mental disorder that has exactly the symptoms you've already described to me—symptoms that the medicine you take is good at controlling. You are not some kind of soulless monster. **(Reality-tests, clarifies, confronts, and reassures)**

Patient: What's going to happen to me? *[tears]*

Therapist: We have better medicines and better therapies than ever before, and I will be here and work with you so that you can improve the quality of your life.

Family Psychoeducation

When supportive treatment is used with higher-functioning patients, environmental manipulation generally is not employed. With more impaired patients, however, the therapist can judiciously intervene in the patient's environment to support continued adaptation and reduce anxiety and stress. A clear example of this approach is family psychoeducation, in which educating the family changes the patient's environment. Teaching the family about the nature of the patient's disorder can help stabilize the family members around the patient in a way that is more supportive of the patient's recovery. Family stabilization is a contrast to the family making the patient the focus of their disappointment, failed expectations, criticism, disbelief, and ignorance. Such family reactions are unlikely to help a patient cope better with chronic illness, and some of these family behaviors, such as high expressed emotion, are clearly associated with exacerbation of illness (Vaughn and Leff 1976). Indeed, short-term family intervention in families with high expressed emotion reduces relapse rates among patients with schizophrenia (Bellack and Mueser 1993).

Personality Disorders

For most therapists, the patients who are most difficult to treat are not the sickest patients (i.e., those with psychotic symptoms and profound impairment of ego functioning) but rather the patients who are highly angry, demanding, suspicious, or dependent (Horowitz and Marmar 1985). Patients with personality disorders use pervasive, maladaptive interpersonal strategies, and their behaviors are sometimes dangerous or frightening. Therefore, these patients can provoke strong negative emotions in people—including psychiatrists, who may avoid treating patients with personality disorders (Lewis and Appleby 1988). The treatability of this class of disorders is contingent on several factors, including disorder severity; the specific diagnosis; the patient's degree of involvement with medical, social, and criminal justice systems; comorbidity; the availability of appropriately trained staff; and the state of scientific knowledge (Adshead 2001).

Clearly, persons administering supportive treatment to such patients must have adequate training or supervision to deal with inevitable countertransference issues, as discussed in Chapter 6, "The Therapeutic Relationship." Nonetheless, supportive psychotherapy is particularly suited to the treatment of most personality disorders, because this therapy focuses on increasing self-esteem and adaptive skills while developing and maintaining a strong therapeutic alliance. As described in Chapter 3, "Assessment, Case Formulation, and Goal Setting," the psychiatrist must conduct an assessment of the patient that allows for a case formulation, including an explication of ego functioning, adaptive skills, object relations, and defensive operations. In certain clusters of personality disorders, patients appear to make greater use of particular groups of maladaptive defenses and defensive behaviors. For example, in the treatment of patients with avoidant personality disorder, a major focus is on getting the patient to develop skills to overcome passivity and fears of rejection. In contrast, in the treatment of patients with narcissistic personality disorder, the focus is on addressing and reducing uses of externalization and criticism. The clinician decides at what point to use more containing, anxiety-reducing supportive technique and when to use expressive technique.

Identifying comorbid mood and anxiety disorders is important in patients with personality disorders. In contrast to earlier concerns that medicating patients would deprive them of the motivation for engagement in treatment, today it is recognized that judicious pharmacological treatment of comorbid depression and anxiety disorders generally acts synergistically with the patients' attempts to learn and master new adaptive skills. In depressed patients, pharmacotherapy reduces Cluster C personality pathology—in particular, harm avoidance, which is associated with poor social function (Hellerstein et al. 2000; Kool et al. 2003; Peselow et al. 1994). When patients are less anxious or less depressed, they are more willing to explore new strategies and may be better able to do so (see Chapter 3 for an evaluation of a patient with major depressive disorder).

In a review of the effectiveness of psychotherapies for personality disorder, Perry et al. (1999) found that all studies of active psychotherapies reported positive outcomes at termination and follow-up. In addition, patients receiving treatment have an accelerated rate of recovery from personality disorders compared with the natural course of the disorders. Bateman and Fonagy (2000) conducted a systematic review of the evidence for efficacy of psychotherapy in personality disorders. Although psychotherapy was found to be effective, the evidence did not indicate that one form of treatment was superior to another. However, effective treatments were found to have several factors in common, including encouragement of a strong patient-therapist relationship that would allow the therapist to take an active rather than passive stance.

Rosenthal et al. (1999) demonstrated lasting change in interpersonal functioning among patients with Cluster C personality disorders who were treated with 40 sessions of manual-based supportive psychotherapy. In addition, in patients with major depressive and personality disorders (especially Cluster C personality disorders), short-term (16-session) supportive psychotherapy in combination with antidepressant treatment reduced personality pathology compared with antidepressant treatment alone (Kool et al. 2003). Patients with problems of hostile dominance, such as patients with antisocial personality disorder, tend to receive less demonstrable benefit from supportive psychotherapy than patients with other personality disorders (Kool et al. 2003; Woody et al. 1985); however, when patients with antisocial personality disorder have comorbid depression, they may do well. Gerstley et al. (1989) hypothesized that the benefit is related to the patients' having some capacity to form a therapeutic alliance.

In supportive psychotherapy, it has been posited that when transference interpretation does not occur, the character-transforming factor may be the patient's capacity to form an identification with the more benign, accepting attitude of the therapist (Appelbaum and Levy 2002; Pinsker et al. 1991). For example, patients with borderline personality disorder typically must contend with what in structural terms is thought of as a rigid, archaic, and punitive superego. Identification with the therapist may allow the patient to be more tolerant of hateful and shameful aspects of the self.

Holmes (1995) reported on borderline patients' use of the commitment, concern, and attention of the supportive technique during analytic treatment and suggested that the development of secure attachments fostered more autonomous functioning. By discouraging destructive behaviors, the therapist models more appropriate behavior and demonstrates strength and concern for the patient (Appelbaum and Levy 2002). As the patient's injurious behaviors and level of emotional intensity diminish, the patient can identify with the reflective function and mentalizing ability of the therapist. This can help the patient make better sense of his or her own subjective states and mental processes, as well as those of others.

Appelbaum and Levy (2002) pointed out that the supportive therapist strives to establish in the patient an arousal level optimal for learning, fostering a sense of self, and appreciating the consequences of behavior. These factors are not unlike those in successful parenting, as Misch (2000) noted, and help to address ego and adaptive dysfunction in patients with borderline personality disorder. With such patients, the therapist works to create a sense of safety so as to reduce maladaptive defenses, which are typically linked to fears of annihilation, abandonment, and humiliation. Creating a sense of safety can help the patient begin to develop a more integrated sense of self and other in the context of reduced anxiety. Nevertheless, this sense of safety must be created without fostering regression, which can escalate those behaviors that the therapist is trying to address and reduce. Maladaptive or immature defenses, such as regression, denial, or projection, are not supported. As in much of supportive psychotherapy, the therapist tries to maintain a balance of supportive and expressive techniques.

An advance in the treatment of borderline personality disorder was the development of dialectical behavior therapy (DBT), which initially focused on reducing parasuicidal behavior (Linehan 1993; Linehan et al. 1994). Although this practical, multicomponent approach to therapy with borderline patients has been presented as an evolution of cognitive-behavioral therapy, certain of the main components of the treatment are decidedly supportive, in that they directly address ego function and adaptive skills. The open and explicit collaboration between patient and therapist on here-and-now issues in DBT is consistent with the style of supportive therapy. In particular, the use of mindfulness exercises is a direct measure that addresses both ego functioning and adaptive skill in teaching patients to develop intrapsychic distance from overwhelming emotional distress. In addition, DBT makes liberal use of slogans and sayings that reframe patients' isolated experience into shared experiential wisdom and that serve as feedback for validating both subjective states and real responsibility (Palmer 2002). Interestingly, a year-long clinical trial comparing DBT, transference-focused psychotherapy, and supportive psychotherapy demonstrated that those receiving supportive psychotherapy had significant positive changes in depression, anxiety, global functioning, and social adjustment. Compared with the DBT group, the supportive psychotherapy group had significant reductions in anger but less efficacy in reducing suicidality, which is not surprising given the specific focus of DBT on parasuicidal behavior (Clarkin et al. 2007).

Substance Use Disorders

Substance use disorders are among the most common mental disorders (Regier et al. 1990). In the past, most psychiatry residents did not treat patients presenting with substance use disorders unless the patients presented with co-occurring psychiatric disorders (see the section "Co-Occurring Mental Illness and Substance Use Disorders" later in this chapter). Generally, residents learned about withdrawal syndromes and detoxification while working on inpatient psychiatric units that admitted patients with psychiatric disorders or substance-induced mental disorders. In contrast, current residency training in psychiatry involves at least 1 month of full-time clinical work with patients who have substance use disorders; thus, residents must learn about basic psychotherapeutic and medication management of these patients. There are relatively few pharmacotherapies that are effective for substance use disorders, and those pharmacotherapies work best in the context of psychosocial treatment. Therefore, psychotherapy is an important intervention for substance use disorders. Some medications approved for use in substance use disorders are maintenance medications for opioid dependence, such as methadone and buprenorphine (Fudala et al. 2003; Kleber 2003), or for alcohol dependence—either aversive medications such as disulfiram (Fuller et al. 1986) or craving reducers such as naltrexone (O'Malley et al. 1992; Volpicelli et al. 1992).

In the past, individual expressive treatments were the standard intervention for substance use disorders. Over time, it became clear that use of uncovering psychotherapy as a sole mode of treatment for substance use disorders was generally not effective. Other treatment approaches, such as group therapies, pharmacotherapies (e.g., methadone maintenance), and therapeutic communities, became mainstays of addiction treatment. Rounsaville and Carroll (1998) underscored the rationale for supportive psychotherapy when they described the reasons that expressive treatments, when offered as the sole ambulatory treatment, are not well suited to the needs of patients with substance use disorders. In expressive treatments, symptom control and development of coping skills are often not the primary focus. Patients drop out frequently because of a lack of focus on the patient's presenting problem and because patients find the therapist's neutral, abstaining stance anxiety provoking. Today, it is understood that interpretations of addictive behaviors are not sufficient to stop the addictive process and that increasing the patient's anxiety early in the treatment of a substance use disorder is likely to trigger a relapse. Therefore, a therapist should embark on a more uncovering type of treatment only when the patient has established a concrete method for maintaining abstinence or is being treated within a protected environment (Brill 1977; Rosenthal and Westreich 1999).

To conduct psychotherapy with substance-abusing patients, the therapist must understand the psychopharmacology of commonly abused classes of drugs, typical presentations of intoxication and withdrawal, and the natural course of drug effects. The therapist also needs to be familiar with common or street knowledge about the drugs, including slang names and prices (Rounsaville and Carroll 1998). A good working knowledge of the drugs of abuse and the lifestyle of the drug-abusing patient can help the therapist begin to build a therapeutic alliance with the patient.

Supportive psychotherapy with patients who have substance use disorder focuses on helping patients to develop effective coping strategies to control or reduce substance use and stay engaged in treatment. Other important components of treatment are developing and maintaining a strong therapeutic alliance and minimizing the risk of relapse by helping the patient to both reduce and learn to manage anxiety and dysphoria. Because supportive psychotherapy offers a broad and flexible foundation for interventions with patients, work with addicted patients typically includes use of newer, more evidence-based strategies, such as motivational interviewing, relapse prevention, and psychoeducation. General supportive principles are maintained during the course of addiction treatment, even as patient and therapist embark on particular cognitive and behavioral work, such as building cognitive skills. For a patient with substance use disorder, individual supportive psychotherapy is often augmented and supported by the patient's engagement in a 12-step program, group therapy for substance use disorders, and other recovery-oriented therapeutic activities.

Motivational Interviewing

If an individual is not interested in reducing or stopping the use of substances when he or she meets the criteria for a substance use disorder, the person may have a diagnosis but is not yet a patient. People who come into treatment for substance use disorders typically have spent months to years without severe consequences and have experienced the drug use as fun or beneficial. People generally show up for substance abuse treatment only when the consequences of their drug use have become threatening to their relationships, employment, health, freedom, or life. When these people then show up for treatment, most of them have beliefs about their drug use that were constructed when their use appeared to be free of severe negative consequences. In addition, a common belief is that drugs have played an essential role in the individual's ability to cope (Rounsaville and Carroll 1998). In this context, unless the patient sees the substance abuse as a problem and can conceptualize getting along without drug use, setting appropriate treatment goals is difficult.

Rollnick and Miller (1995) described motivational interviewing as a directive, patient-centered intervention that helps patients to explore and resolve their ambivalence about changing. The main principles of motivational interviewing include understanding the patient's view accurately, avoiding or deescalating resistance, and increasing the patient's self-efficacy and perception of the discrepancy between actual and ideal behavior (Miller and Rollnick 1991). Motivational interviewing is explicitly empathic and does not involve a coercive therapist position with respect to the patient's actions about reducing or stopping substance use; the patient might experience such a position as demeaning and damaging to self-esteem. A premise of motivational interviewing is that patients can decide to make changes on the basis of their own shifts in motivation. The techniques of motivational interviewing include listening reflectively and eliciting motivational statements from a patient, examining both sides of the patient's ambivalence, and reducing resistance by monitoring patient readiness and not pushing for change prematurely (Miller and Rollnick 1991). When the patient experiences that the negative consequences of substance use outweigh the positives ones, the so-called decisional balance is tipped in favor of engagement in treatment.

Substantial evidence supports motivational interviewing as an effective intervention for substance use disorders—especially with regard to promoting entry into and engagement in more-intensive substance abuse treatment—even when the technique is used by clinicians who are not substance abuse treatment specialists (Dunn et al. 2001). Therefore, motivational interviewing is a mainstay of supportive treatment of substance use disorders.

Adaptive Skills and Relapse Prevention

The main content of supportive treatment of substance use disorders is the work of achieving and maintaining abstinence from substances of abuse. Patients must learn new strategies that assist them in coping with craving states, negative emotions, general stress, and cues in the environment that serve as high-risk triggers for substance use. Long ago, the proponents of Alcoholics Anonymous identified exposure to the "people, places, and things" associated with alcohol use as a primer to relapse. A commonly heard maxim is that stopping the use of drugs is relatively easy, but remaining drug-free is hard. The specific adaptive skills that must be learned in addiction recovery are 1) identifying high-risk situations and cues, 2) anticipating exposure to these situations and cues, and 3) developing alternative strategies for coping when exposed to these situations.

Relapse prevention involves a formal set of cognitive-behavioral approaches to maintaining abstinence that are easily woven into supportive treatment. In relapse prevention, a systematic effort is made to identify the patient's specific relapse triggers and to devise and have the patient practice alternative behaviors and coping skills to deal with these triggers, such as refusal skills for when the patient is offered the target substance (Marlatt and Gordon 1985). However, identification of risky situations and development of coping skills to address these situations can also be done in a less structured fashion in supportive and supportive-expressive psychotherapy (Luborsky 1984). In any case, anticipatory guidance, encouragement, and reassurance are key supportive techniques that are used when identifying and rehearsing skills to cope with an expected situation. The therapist works to establish achievable intermediate goals, which help to reduce the risk of failure and of further damage to the patient's self-esteem. When the patient reports that he or she has successfully negotiated some element of a high-risk situation, therapist praise related to the patient's goals is meaningful and reinforces the improvement in adaptive skills. The patient should already have experienced some increase in self-esteem through an experience of competence in achieving a life skill. If the patient tries and does not succeed, some praise is indicated, because the patient tried to implement the adaptive skill. After some problem solving together, the therapist encourages the patient to try the skill again, and reassures him or her about doing so. Thus, progress in executing new skills may be incremental, and the therapist offers measured but increasingly intense praise and positive feedback for each successive goal met.

Because a dysphoric mood is the most frequently reported antecedent of relapse, the supportive treatment of substance use disorders also must focus on building adaptive skills for coping with negative or painful mood states (Marlatt and Gordon 1980). Substance-abusing individuals often have a difficult time differentiating mood states into specific affects, in part perhaps because they use the drugs to self-medicate dysphoria, rather than developing psychological means to cope with the painful affects (Keller et al. 1995; Khantzian 1985). Therefore, therapists need to help patients with substance use disorder begin to reduce alexithymia in distinguishing one feeling from another. As Misch (2000) described, the ability to identify and label feelings makes it easier to reflect on them and communicate about feelings to others. If the patient cannot notice and discriminate feelings, he or she cannot make clear connections between those feelings and the thoughts, behaviors, or events linked to drug use. For example, if patients cannot recognize when they are irritable and sad, they will not be able to connect either state to the automatic thoughts that they generate in response (e.g., "I'm feeling irritated, so I must get a bottle"). The ability to label feelings is essential for developing appropriate adaptive skills to manage painful affects. As patients begin to identify these feelings, they experience—in spite of increased awareness of negative affect—an increase in self-esteem that comes from mastery of the internal environment. The affects begin to be reframed as useful tools in identifying risky states that set patients up for relapse.

Psychoeducation

In the area of substance use disorders, education efforts focus on teaching patients about different classes of abused drugs, psychological and physical effects of drugs, dangers of chronic abuse, the fact that drugs may be used to self-medicate, and a disease model of addiction. Most cultures implicitly or explicitly operate out of a moral model of substance abuse and addiction, which attributes the irresponsible or criminal behavior of the addicted individual to his or her bad character. In contrast, the unitary disease concept of addiction, variously attributed to Alcoholics Anonymous (1976) or Jellinek (1952), stresses that addiction is a chronic, relapsing, and progressive illness. Furthermore, the advocates of the disease concept thought it was a mistake to think of alcoholism as a symptom of another disorder, such that if an underlying conflict were resolved in expressive treatment, the patient would stop drinking (Rosenthal and Westreich 1999). Jellinek's approach to alcoholism was not actually so reductionistic; he in fact described several typologies, which differed regarding onset, severity, pattern, and chronicity of use. Nonetheless, the psychotherapeutic utility of this heuristic approach is that it increases self-esteem by offering the patient a diagnosis rather than blame, helps the patient to cope better with shame (given that most patients presume that the moral model explains their own behavior), and offers another framework in which to foster a therapeutic alliance.

The following vignette illustrates the use of psychoeducation with a substance-abusing patient (see Vignette 6 on the DVD).

▶ **Vignette 6:**
Substance Use Disorder

Mr. Waters is a 28-year-old single man who studied structural engineering in college but is currently unemployed, having been fired from his most recent of a string of jobs over the last few years, since he began using cocaine. He typically gets caught up in cocaine bingeing and fails to show up or notify his place of employment, with predictable results. He was living with his younger sister, her husband, and their 2-year-old daughter but was told to leave when he returned after a 3-day cocaine binge. He comes to the session full of regret and self-recrimination, a strong sense of the moral failure he has been given as feedback from both employers and family, and hopelessness.

Other cases might rely more strongly on motivational interviewing techniques in the early phases (including nonjudgmental feedback to help the patient connect cause and effect) and thus assist him in deciding that his substance dependence isn't worth what it costs in his life. In this session, the therapist instead uses psychoeducation to address the patient's denial and use of a moral model to explain his addictive behavior. Because the moral model is intrinsically disempowering, which decreases self-esteem, the objective is that the patient understand the disease concept and that the loss of control is an inherent quality of substance dependence. The patient may then feel more empowered to make decisions that incorporate that reality, rather than channeling his energy into self-blaming and unfruitful behavior that typically precedes or sustains a relapse.

▶ **Vignette 6:**
Substance Use Disorder *(continued)*

Mr. Waters: I can't stop…the crack. I got thrown out of the house.…
I got no job, I got no money, I got no girl, I got nothing…except
crack. I've blown up my life. *[sighs, looks at therapist]* Maybe
they're right. Maybe I'm just no good. *[looks down, shakes head,
tears]* **(Attributes his drug-related losses and maladaptive behavior to being a bad person)**

Therapist: I know the pain you're in right now makes you want to just
blame yourself. And you've got a lot of reasons to feel bad right
now. But can I ask you to consider your intentions for just a moment? It's important, but it will take a bit of reflection. **(Empathically focuses patient away from self-blame to cognition)**

Mr. Waters: OK.

Therapist: If you knew then what you know now—that your use results in the way your life is right now and the way you feel now—
would you have done it anyway? **(Clarification)**

Mr. Waters: Nah, don't think so. No, of course not.… I wouldn't have
done this…if I had known.… No! *[angry]* **(Takes rational position)**

Therapist: So, what I'm saying to you is that your situation is predictable. This is what happens to people who become addicted to
crack. Addiction is like a runaway train: once you get on board,
you don't necessarily go where you want the train to go. You go
where the train takes you. **(Generalizes to others who have the
same well-described problem, offers teaching metaphor)**

Mr. Waters: Yeah, but I'm the one who keeps doing it.… I'm the one
who started this up.… I'm the one who doesn't stop. Like there's
something's wrong with me! I'm stupid! **(Retreats to moral
model explanation, holds on to denial of loss of control)**

Therapist: Well, I guess blaming yourself gives you some sense that
you're still in control of this situation and that it's OK, when
clearly it's not!

Mr. Waters: I don't understand.

Therapist: Well, let me put it this way: If you were stupid and couldn't
learn, then that would explain the situation, but you're not stupid. You studied engineering successfully in college. Right?
**(Confronts distortion in self-description, builds alliance
through demonstrating knowledge of patient's personal history)**

Mr. Waters: Yeah, OK. So, I'm not stupid-stupid, but I've done such
stupid stuff! *[scowls]* Maybe my sister is right; maybe I'm just
weak and selfish. **(Acknowledges distortion, but retreats to a
different form of self-blame)**

> ▶ **Vignette 6:**
> **Substance Use Disorder** *(continued)*

Therapist: So you just told me that if you knew then what you know now, you would not have made the same choices, and that now you're in a position where you can't stop. That's why we call it a disease. Loss of control comes with the territory; it's part of the disease. Drugs are powerful that way. *(Confronts denial, which is maladaptive for this patient; offers a different explanation)*

Mr. Waters: I understand what you're saying, Doc, but you might be saying this just to make me feel better—and that's fine—but I got the rest of the world telling me I'm a waste of skin. Hey, I appreciate that, but…

Therapist: Let me show you something. These are the criteria for substance dependence in DSM. What you see here is that loss of control is one of the major symptoms. Right? *[opens DSM-IV-TR to criteria for substance dependence and points to the text while reading out loud]* "The substance is often taken in larger amounts or over a longer period than was intended. There is a persistent desire or unsuccessful efforts to cut down or control substance use" [American Psychiatric Association 2000, p. 197]. *(Uses props, if necessary, to concretize the ideas and demonstrate expertise)*

Mr. Waters: Huh. So I've tried so many times to just do only some drugs, but I always spend everything I have. *(Recognizes own loss of control, becomes sad)*

Therapist: So, maybe initially when you started, you made the mistake of thinking that you could get away with just using, but that was a long time ago. Things are a little different now. What you have now is called a disorder. Addiction and alcoholism are things that run in families. They are inherited. The risk is inherited, and drug problems are very similar. *(Supports patient's understanding with clarification, normalizing, rationalizing, and new knowledge)*

Mr. Waters: My dad was alcoholic. So was my uncle. I think that's what killed my uncle. *(Confirms understanding that his problems are more than just about willpower)*

Therapist: So, that's my point…. It's not your fault—but maybe now you understand that you and I must work together in order to help you fight this disease. *(Sides with the patient against the disease, supports the need for collaboration)*

Mr. Waters: Aw, man, it just seems impossible. Do you think I really can get help with this? *(Elicits reassurance)*

Therapist: I know it seems that way now, particularly when you recognize your own loss of control, but this is a very common experience for people who are in the early stages or in the beginnings of recovery. But those who stay with treatments tend to have better outcomes than those who don't stay with treatments. *(Offers empathic reassurance based on expert knowledge, normalizing)*

▶ **Vignette 6:**
Substance Use Disorder *(continued)*

Mr. Waters: I hope you're right.

Therapist: I know right now it seems like there's a very long way to go.... This is going to be difficult, but addiction is a treatable illness, like many other chronic illnesses. We don't have a cure for diabetes. We don't have a cure for hypertension. But people are able to recover from the more severe forms of the illness.... Even with the illness being out of control, they can go on to have better lives. *(Expert opinion, normalizing, and offering reassurance)*

Co-Occurring Mental Illness and Substance Use Disorders

About half the population with severe mental disorders is affected by substance abuse or dependence (Regier et al. 1990). Clinical samples of psychiatric patients often have higher-than-usual rates of alcohol use disorders and other substance use disorders (Fernandez-Pol et al. 1988; Fischer et al. 1975; Galanter et al. 1988; Richard et al. 1985). In the National Comorbidity Survey, Kessler et al. (1994) found that of the population who had psychosis or mania or who needed hospitalization for a mental disorder in a 12-month period, almost 90% met the criteria for three or more lifetime alcohol or drug use disorders or mental disorders.

Co-occurrence of mental illness and substance use disorders has a negative effect on the trajectory of and recovery from both disorders (Rosenthal and Westreich 1999). Because patients with substance use disorders and schizophrenia are difficult to engage in treatment, supportive psychotherapy, with its focus on building and maintaining a therapeutic alliance, is a good treatment approach for this population (Carey et al. 1996; Lehman et al. 1993). Supportive treatment for those with both disorders integrates the techniques that are useful for each problem, as delineated in the sections "Severe Mental Illness" and "Substance Use Disorders" earlier in this chapter. Improving adaptive skills by increasing competence in basic conversational and recreational skills, using medication and symptom management, and using relapse prevention for negotiating situations likely to trigger relapse to substance abuse are all generally needed to treat co-occurring substance use disorders and mental illness. Implementing these interventions has a beneficial effect on treatment retention and substance use in patients with psychotic illness and substance use disorders (Ho et al. 1999). Multiple studies have shown that psychosocial treatment that integrates psychiatric and addiction treatment components leads to better retention and better outcome among patients with severe mental illness and substance use disorders (Drake et al. 2001; Hellerstein et al. 1995).

Additional factors that work in concert with individual supportive treatment are support for patient involvement in 12-step programs (especially programs that are less likely to reduce self-esteem, such as "double trouble" or "dual recovery" groups) and family psychoeducation. In addition to praise, support for access to concrete services, socialization, recreation, and other opportunities can serve as positive reinforcement for attendance and may support the development of a therapeutic alliance and the engagement of patients in treatment (Rosenthal et al. 2000).

Psychoeducation

In the context of supportive treatment, patients with substance use disorders and mental illness should be given information about both classes of disorders. Like other supportive techniques, psychoeducation must be formulated in the context of the therapist's appraisal of the patient's capacity to make use of the information in a way that supports ego function or adaptive skills. For example, when a patient with a severe mental illness learns that he or she has another chronic illness such as substance dependence, this knowledge can become a factor in his or her demoralization (Rosenthal and Westreich 1999). The therapist teaches about both the substance dependence and the mental illness: their symptoms, treatment, and natural history. Patients are encouraged to discuss their own symptoms and their own history of treatment responsiveness and to attempt to understand what role their substance abuse may have played in either relieving or exacerbating psychotic, mood, and anxiety symptoms.

Most patients with co-occurring substance use disorders and severe mental disorders who come into contact with treatment systems are not motivated to stop the use of substances. With these patients, motivational interviewing techniques can be useful within the context of supportive psychotherapy (Ziedonis and Fisher 1996; Ziedonis and Trudeau 1997). The process of recovery in patients with comorbid substance use disorders and mental disorders is not linear, and exacerbation of both disorders is episodic. Patients may cycle repeatedly through different phases of treatment—engagement, active treatment, maintenance, relapse, and then reengagement. When patients come back into contact with treating clinicians after a relapse, they may be in an earlier motivational stage; they may even be in denial that a substance abuse problem exists (Prochaska and DiClemente 1984). Motivational techniques, which are traditionally used at the beginning of therapy to engage patients with substance use disorder in treatment, are thus used as a continuing component of supportive treatment for patients with co-occurring substance use disorders and severe mental illness. This approach is needed because patients cycle between motivational levels, with the various flare-ups of substance use disorders and other mental illness over time (Rosenthal and Westreich 1999). The time frame of recovery from substance use disorders is longer for patients with dual diagnoses than for patients without comorbid severe mental disorders. If a patient remains in treatment, however, reduction in severity of both disorders is a realistic prospect (Drake et al. 1993; Hellerstein et al. 1995).

Conclusion

Supportive psychotherapy provides a broad basic platform for psychotherapeutic intervention; therefore, treatment strategies and approaches such as motivational interviewing, psychoeducation, and relapse prevention, which are typically associated with specific clinical subpopulations, can be readily implemented in the context of a supportive treatment. In patients with personality disorders, supportive psychotherapy has beneficial impact and can serve as a natural platform for integrating other treatment strategies (e.g., using dialectical behavior therapy for patients with borderline personality disorder). In populations such as those with co-occurring substance use and other mental disorders, the alliance-building strategies of supportive psychotherapy plus motivational techniques can be applied over time to help maintain the patient's engagement in treatment through cycles of relapse and recovery.

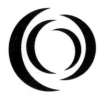

9

Evaluating Competence and Outcome Research

The Accreditation Council for Graduate Medical Education (ACGME) defined six areas of competence for medical trainees: 1) patient care, 2) medical knowledge, 3) practice-based learning and improvement, 4) interpersonal and communication skills, 5) professionalism, and 6) systems-based practice (ACGME Outcomes Project 2000). Although outlining and describing areas of competence are within grasp at the present time, the tasks of defining, evaluating, and measuring competence of trainees are more complex. Development of measurement tools and their application to specific areas of competence is under way but still in an early stage. The ACGME suggested a dozen methods of measuring competence. These methods, which the ACGME labeled "the Toolbox," include various types of written, oral, and clinical examinations; a combined assessment approach of patient, family, supervisors, and others; record reviews; portfolios and case logs; simulations, models, and use of standardized patients; and evaluation of live or recorded performance. The Residency Review Committee for Psychiatry chose five types of psychotherapy in which residents in psychiatry must be certified as competent by their training programs, but a few years later decreased this requirement to three types: supportive, psychodynamic, and cognitive-behavioral psychotherapies (ACGME 2007). In this chapter, we outline our approach to evaluating competence of psychiatry trainees in one of these three psychotherapies—namely, supportive psychotherapy.

The definition of *competence* is a major issue that needs to be addressed. An acceptable definition of *competent* is "having requisite or adequate ability or qualities" (*Merriam-Webster's Collegiate Dictionary*, 11th Edition). Epstein and Hundert (2002) defined *professional competence* as "the habitual and judicious use of communication, knowledge, technical skills, clinical reasoning, emotions, values, and reflection in daily practice for the benefit of the individual and community being served" (p. 226). In assessments of psychotherapy trainees, supervisors should look for competence, not a high level of expertise (Manring et al. 2003).

When addressing a resident's competence, it is necessary to define what will be assessed and the method or methods of assessment. The evaluation process should be educational and promote resident learning. Professional competence can be conceptualized as a continuum of levels of ability or skill, from beginner to competent to expert. A trainee would be expected to be competent and thus be at the middle of this continuum.

Psychotherapy Supervision

Assessment of residents' competence in psychotherapy is an ongoing process in many residency programs. In the main, evaluations of residents are performed by clinical supervisors during the process of psychotherapy supervision and are formally discussed with the residents one or more times a year.

Clinical supervision, as well as more formal seminars and classroom teaching, has long been a part of psychotherapy training. Seminars and classroom approaches generally consist of reading courses, in which psychotherapy theory and practice are taught, and clinical case seminars, which focus on evaluation, case formulation, diagnosis, and ongoing psychotherapy. Many training programs in psychiatry have established traditions of intensive individual supervision of residents, particularly in long-term expressive (exploratory) psychotherapy. The process of supervision may vary from one program to another but generally involves the following:

1. Presentation of the case by the resident
2. Discussion of the diagnosis, case formulation, goals, and treatment plan
3. Ongoing summary of sessions by the resident, using an informal recall-and-summary approach, process notes, video recordings, or a combination of these approaches
4. Discussion of the psychotherapy process, including resistance, dysfunctional thinking, defenses, affect, and therapist interventions, as well as dynamics, genetics, psychological structure, cognitive-behavioral issues, and the therapeutic relationship (transference, countertransference, and the therapeutic alliance)

The supervisor has traditionally evaluated the resident's work by noting how well the resident performs the tasks listed above, as well as assessing other areas such as the ability to listen and relate to the patient in an empathic manner. The evaluation process by the supervisor is ongoing, but formal evaluations are generally performed once or twice a year or more. The formal evaluations are based on material discussed by the trainee through the use of process notes. Traditionally, the entire process has been somewhat informal and rarely standardized. In this chapter, we propose a standardized evaluation approach, one based on the use of video recordings during an ongoing course of psychotherapy.

Assessment

Focus

Assessment of competence in supportive psychotherapy should be evaluated within the broader context of general psychotherapy. The assessment should encompass skills of, attitudes toward, and knowledge about general psychotherapy and the more specific approach of supportive psychotherapy. General psychotherapy skills, as described by the American Association of Directors of Psychiatric Residency Training (AADPRT) Psychotherapy Task Force (2000), include establishing and maintaining boundaries and the therapeutic alliance, listening, addressing emotions, understanding, using supervision, dealing with resistances and defenses, and applying intervention techniques. Beitman and Yue (1999) described a similar set of skills, which they called core psychotherapy skills. They included other skills, such as identifying patterns and implementing strategies for change. The AADPRT Psychotherapy Task Force also developed psychotherapy competencies for the five psychotherapies originally mandated by the Residency Review Committee for Psychiatry, including supportive psychotherapy. Table 9–1 includes the complete list of AADPRT competencies for supportive psychotherapy (Pinsker et al. 2001).

The supportive psychotherapy competencies are divided into knowledge about, skills of, and attitudes toward supportive psychotherapy. The knowledge category encompasses knowledge about objectives, the patient-therapist relationship, and indications and contraindications for supportive psychotherapy. The skills section contains 15 items, including the ability to maintain a therapeutic alliance, the ability to use appropriate interventions, and the ability to establish treatment goals. The attitudes section includes an empathic, respectful, nonjudgmental approach and sensitivity to sociocultural, socioeconomic, and educational issues.

Table 9–1. American Association of Directors of Psychiatric Residency Training competencies for supportive psychotherapy

Knowledge
1. The resident will demonstrate knowledge that the principal objectives of supportive therapy are to maintain or improve the patient's self-esteem, minimize or prevent recurrence of symptoms, and maximize the patient's adaptive capacities.
2. The resident will demonstrate understanding that the practice of supportive therapy is commonly used in many therapeutic encounters.
3. The resident will demonstrate knowledge that the patient-therapist relationship is of paramount importance.
4. The resident will demonstrate knowledge of indications and contraindications for supportive therapy.
5. The resident will demonstrate understanding that continued education in supportive therapy is necessary for further skill development.

Skills
1. The resident will be able to establish and maintain a therapeutic alliance.
2. The resident will be able to establish treatment goals.
3. The resident will be able to interact in a direct and nonthreatening manner.
4. The resident will be able to be responsive to the patient and give feedback and advice when appropriate.
5. The resident will demonstrate the ability to understand the patient as a unique individual within his or her family and sociocultural community.
6. The resident will be able to determine which interventions are in the best interest of the patient and will exercise caution about basing interventions on his or her own beliefs and values.
7. The resident will be able to recognize and identify affects in the patient and himself or herself.
8. The resident will be able to confront in a collaborative manner behaviors that are dangerous or damaging to the patient.
9. The resident will be able to provide reassurance to reduce symptoms, improve morale and adaptation, and prevent relapse.
10. The resident will be able to support, promote, and recognize the patient's ability to achieve goals that will promote his or her well-being.
11. The resident will be able to provide strategies to manage problems with affect regulation, thought disorders, and impaired reality-testing.
12. The resident will be able to provide education and advice about the patient's psychiatric condition, treatment, and adaptation while being sensitive to specific community systems of care and sociocultural issues.
13. The resident will be able to demonstrate that in the care of patients with chronic disorders, attention should be directed to adaptive skills, relationships, morale, and potential sources of anxiety or worry.
14. The resident will be able to assist the patient in developing skills for self-assessment.

Table 9–1.   American Association of Directors of Psychiatric
Residency Training competencies for supportive
psychotherapy *(continued)*

---

15. The resident will be able to seek appropriate consultation and/or referral
for specialized treatment.

Attitudes
1. The resident will be empathic, respectful, curious, open, nonjudgmental,
collaborative, and able to tolerate ambiguity and display confidence in the
efficacy of supportive therapy.
2. The resident will be sensitive to sociocultural, socioeconomic, and
educational issues that arise in the therapeutic relationship.
3. The resident will be open to audiotaping, videotaping, or direct
observation of treatment sessions.

Source.   Pinsker et al. 2001.

Method

Assessment of a trainee's competence in supportive psychotherapy can
be accomplished using a number of different methodologies, including
administration of written and/or oral examinations that test the resident's
knowledge base, use of simulated patients reading from standardized
scripts, the request that the resident respond to a patient vignette using a
supportive approach, and a supervisor's evaluation of a resident perform-
ing supportive psychotherapy. We have found that supervisor evaluations
of ongoing, video-recorded psychotherapy sessions are the best method
of teaching and evaluating residents. Video-recorded sessions enable the
supervisor or resident evaluator to observe the conduct of psychotherapy
directly. The more traditional method of summarizing a session or working from process notes is less likely to convey what actually occurred in a
psychotherapy session, even under the best of circumstances. The availability of video recordings opens the process of psychotherapy to an outside observer and makes evaluation of therapy more objective.

Evaluation of video-recorded supportive psychotherapy sessions
should begin with the resident's assessment of the patient and should
continue throughout a patient's psychotherapy. Each supervision session
should begin with a brief summary by the resident, followed by a review
of the video recording. Because an entire video recording is likely too
lengthy for review in a supervisory hour, the supervisor and resident must
decide which segments to review. The choice of video segments for viewing can be made on the basis of the resident's summary, which may point
to areas of difficulty or significance. A formal written evaluation of the
resident by the supervisor should be completed at least twice a year. This

evaluation should be educative and be based on the supervisory work preceding the formal evaluation. The supervisor should provide the resident with verbal feedback on a regular basis.

Having trainees view recordings of psychotherapy sessions conducted by others essentially replaces a supervisory experience and can be used to assess the trainee's knowledge level, which cannot always be equated with skill. This procedure allows for discussion of techniques and of the broad range of possible therapeutic interventions.

A number of questions have been raised about the feasibility of using video recordings of psychotherapy for supervision. Difficulties cited include the cost and maintenance of the equipment and the ability of residents to operate the recording equipment. The cost of video equipment has decreased in recent years, enabling many training programs to offer video recording to residents. Also, video equipment has become easy to operate, and residents are able to make good recordings. Therefore, it seems feasible for residency programs to provide video equipment for residency training in psychotherapy.

In the event that video equipment cannot be provided by the institution, it would not be unreasonable to require each trainee to provide his or her own camera. After all, training programs generally do not provide each resident with textbooks. The main purpose of recording is not to have a high-quality picture but rather an understandable audio that runs without attention from the therapist for the entire session.

Some residency programs may not be ready to begin with evaluations involving video. The evaluation form presented in the next section of this chapter can be used to evaluate a trainee reporting on psychotherapy sessions from process notes. Another approach would be to present a video recording or written material from a supportive psychotherapy session and ask the resident questions about the treatment plan, case formulation, goals, technique, alliance, and so on. In addition, the resident could be asked to respond to the patient's complaints using a supportive psychotherapy approach.

Assessment Instrument

The AADPRT supportive psychotherapy competencies provided the basis for our development of a rating form to be used as a measure of a resident's competence in supportive psychotherapy. Our form (Figure 9–1) does not include all the items on the AADPRT list of competencies because it would not be practical or reasonable for training programs to use lengthy evaluation forms for three different psychotherapies. In addition, we modified or combined some items with other items from the supportive psychotherapy and general psychotherapy competencies.

The evaluation form covers three areas: knowledge, attitudes, and skills. For example, the first item in the knowledge and attitudes section is the following: "The resident demonstrates knowledge that the principal objectives of supportive psychotherapy are to maintain or improve the patient's self-esteem, ameliorate or prevent recurrence of symptoms, improve psychological or ego functioning, and enhance adaptive capacities." The rating is on a Likert scale of 0–5 (0=can't say, 1=unsatisfactory, 2=approaching competence, 3=competent, 4=competent plus, 5=expert). In the skills section, item 1 is the following: "The resident is able to establish and maintain a positive therapeutic alliance and interact with the patient in an empathic, respectful, direct, responsive, nonthreatening manner." An item taken from general psychotherapy competencies, placed in the knowledge and attitudes section (item 5), is worded thus: "The resident understands that appropriate boundaries (e.g., time, outside agencies and relationships, confidentiality, and professional attitude) must be established and maintained."

The advantages of this evaluation form are that it can be scored and that it also includes space for the supervisor's comments. The final score is calculated by dividing the number of questions scored into the total score. An average score of 3 or better suggests that the resident has demonstrated competence in supportive psychotherapy. In addition, the supervisor should write some overall comments about the resident, including the resident's strengths and overall performance, areas needing further work, and the resident's ability to work in and use supervision. The supervisor should discuss the evaluation with the resident in a way that is supportive and promotes the resident's education.

To standardize the evaluation of competence in supportive psychotherapy, conferences in which supportive psychotherapy supervisors discuss the supervisory and evaluation processes would be important. One method of achieving reliability would be to have groups of supervisors rate supportive psychotherapy video recordings and then discuss their ratings. Discussions would be directed at reaching a consensus in the evaluation ratings. This approach has been used in psychotherapy research to measure therapist adherence to manual-based forms of psychotherapy (Waltz et al. 1993).

From 2006 to 2010, supervisors in the Beth Israel Medical Center Psychotherapy Training Program rated 39 residents on their supportive psychotherapy work using the Resident Evaluation for Competence in Supportive Psychotherapy. We have found that the vast majority of residents were rated as competent or better. More important, the form served as a useful supportive psychotherapy evaluation guide for both residents and supervisors, and the supervisors found the form to be useful and easy to use.

Resident Evaluation for Competence in Supportive Psychotherapy

Resident _____ Supervisor _____

Date _____ Period _____

Instructions: Please evaluate the resident's performance on the following items by entering the appropriate number on the scoring line after each item.

Can't say	Unsatisfactory	Approaching competence	Competent	Competent plus	Expert
0	1	2	3	4	5

Knowledge and attitudes   Score

1. The resident demonstrates knowledge that the principal objectives of supportive psychotherapy are to maintain or improve the patient's self-esteem, ameliorate or prevent recurrence of symptoms, improve psychological or ego functioning, and enhance adaptive capacities. _____

2. The resident understands that supportive therapy is dynamically based and is part of a continuum ranging from supportive to expressive psychotherapy. _____

3. The resident demonstrates knowledge that the patient-therapist relationship is of paramount importance and is not addressed unless it is negative. _____

4. The resident demonstrates knowledge of indications and contraindications for supportive psychotherapy. _____

5. The resident understands that appropriate boundaries (e.g., time, outside agencies and relationships, confidentiality, professional attitude) must be established and maintained. _____

Skills   Score

1. The resident is able to establish and maintain a positive therapeutic alliance and interact with the patient in an empathic, respectful, direct, responsive, and nonthreatening manner. _____

2. The resident relates to the patient in a conversational manner (i.e., does not interrogate or engage in passive listening). _____

3. The resident is able to establish realistic and appropriate treatment goals. _____

4. The resident uses supportive therapy interventions (clarification, confrontation, interpretation, advice, reassurance, encouragement, praise, rationalization, reframing) in an appropriate and timely manner. _____

5. The resident is able to respect and strengthen adaptive defenses, distinguish between adaptive and maladaptive defenses, and work to minimize anxiety in an appropriate and timely manner. _____

6. The resident provides education about the patient's psychiatric condition and medication, and if necessary, about community systems of care and ancillary treatments. _____

Figure 9–1. Resident Evaluation for Competence in Supportive Psychotherapy.

7. The resident focuses on the patient's present-day life while not ignoring the past and consistently works at improving self-esteem, promoting adaptation and ego functions, and ameliorating symptoms. ____

Total score: ____

Divided by number of items scored: ____ = ____

Supervisor's comments *(include comments on overall performance, strengths, areas needing further work, and the ability to work in and use supervision):*

_____

_____

_____

_____

Resident's signature _____
(This evaluation was discussed with me.)

Supervisor's signature_____

Evaluation based on *(check all that apply)*
Weekly supervision ____　Review of psychotherapy video ____
Review of psychotherapy notes ____

Figure 9–1. Resident Evaluation for Competence in Supportive Psychotherapy. *(continued)*

Outcome Research

Results from a limited number of controlled clinical trials of supportive psychotherapy have been reported. In this section, we discuss some early uncontrolled studies and some more recent controlled trials that address the efficacy of supportive psychotherapy.

Menninger Psychotherapy Research Project

The psychotherapy research project of the Menninger Foundation was an important early study comparing supportive and expressive psychotherapy with psychoanalysis. Wallerstein (1986, 1989) studied the treatment, clinical course, and posttreatment follow-up of 42 inpatients at the Menninger Foundation. Findings included the following: psychoanalysis produced more limited outcomes than predicted, whereas psychotherapy including supportive psychotherapy often achieved more than predicted; all the treatments became more supportive during the course of therapy;

and supportive interventions accounted for more of the change in outcome. This study took a naturalistic approach, without control subjects or random assignment of subjects, but it was noteworthy in calling attention to the possible efficacy of supportive psychotherapy.

Schizophrenia Studies

In a National Institute of Mental Health study, patients with schizophrenia were treated for 2 years with either exploratory, insight-oriented psychotherapy three times a week or the control therapy (called reality-adaptive, supportive psychotherapy) once a week. Results provided clear evidence of a better outcome for patients treated with the supportive psychotherapy (Gunderson et al. 1984; Stanton et al. 1984). All patients were maintained on their usual medications throughout the study.

In another study, patients with schizophrenia were randomly assigned to supportive psychotherapy or family treatment (Rea et al. 1991). Patients were treated for 9 months and followed for 2 years. Supportive psychotherapy consisted of medication case management, crisis intervention, and education about schizophrenia, whereas family treatment involved problem-solving therapy and communication skills training. Patients in supportive treatment had significant improvement in coping style compared with patients in family therapy. However, the two treatment groups were not at comparable levels of coping skills, and this fact was not considered in the statistical analysis.

Hogarty et al. (1997) stated that supportive psychotherapy fares less well compared with other psychosocial approaches, such as family psychoeducation, skills training, or role therapy. However, defining *supportive psychotherapy* as not including psychoeducation, skills training, or role therapy approaches is problematic because most therapists practicing supportive psychotherapy commonly employ these approaches. Other psychotherapy approaches with patients who have schizophrenia include social skills training, which may be enhanced with amplified skills training in the community (Glynn et al. 2002; Liberman et al. 1998).

Depressive Disorder Studies

In the National Institute of Mental Health Treatment of Depression Collaborative Research Program, two psychotherapies (cognitive-behavioral therapy and interpersonal therapy) were compared with an antidepressant (imipramine)–clinical management condition and a control condition consisting of drug placebo and clinical management (Elkin 1994; Elkin et al. 1989; Imber et al. 1990). The clinical management was a low-level supportive psychotherapy approach. The two psychotherapies were found to be efficacious but not significantly different from the placebo–clinical management condition on measures of depressive symptoms and overall functioning.

Thompson and Gallagher (1985) studied 30 outpatients ranging in age from 60 to 81 years. Patients were randomly assigned to a 16-week treatment with cognitive therapy, behavior treatment, or supportive psychotherapy. Improvement was similar across the three treatment conditions at termination, but at 1-year follow-up, more of the patients in supportive psychotherapy received a diagnosis of depression. Unfortunately, the small number of patients in each treatment group and the type of supportive psychotherapy used make these findings of limited value.

In a randomized clinical trial involving 100 adolescents with depression, Renaud et al. (1998) compared cognitive, family, and supportive psychotherapies and found that rapid responders to therapy had better outcomes at 1-year follow-up and better scores on some measures at 2-year follow-up. The investigators concluded that their findings suggest that patients with milder forms of depression may benefit from initial supportive psychotherapy or short trials of more specialized types of psychotherapy.

Maina et al. (2005) completed a randomized controlled trial comparing brief dynamic therapy with supportive psychotherapy in treating patients with minor depressive disorders. Both therapies showed significant improvement in comparison with nontreated control subjects, but brief dynamic therapy was more effective at follow-up evaluation.

In a mega-analysis involving patients with major depression, de Maat et al. (2008) compared short-term psychodynamic supportive psychotherapy with antidepressant treatment and also with combined psychotherapy and medication. The results of the mega-analysis indicated that combined therapy is more efficacious than pharmacotherapy alone, and that psychotherapy alone and pharmacotherapy alone seem equally efficacious.

Kocsis et al. (2009) compared a cognitive-behavioral analysis system of psychotherapy with brief supportive psychotherapy in their ability to augment antidepressant nonresponse in patients with chronic depression. Although 37.5% of subjects experienced partial response or remission, neither form of adjunctive psychotherapy improved outcome compared with a flexible, individualized pharmacotherapy regimen alone.

Anxiety Disorder Studies

Systematic hierarchical desensitization was compared with supportive psychotherapy in a 26-week treatment trial involving patients with various types of phobias (Klein et al. 1983). Both treatments performed well, and no difference was found between the two approaches. The authors speculated that for individuals with phobia, psychotherapy serves as an instigator of corrective activity outside the formal session by maintaining exposure in vivo. In another study, patients with phobias and panic attacks received either imipramine plus behavior therapy or imipramine plus supportive psychotherapy (Zitrin et al. 1978). The majority of patients showed moderate to marked improvement, and there was no difference between behavior therapy and supportive psychotherapy in terms of improvement rates.

In a study of social anxiety disorder (phobia), Alstrom et al. (1984) found that supportive psychotherapy and prolonged exposure therapy were equally effective. Herbert et al. (2009) compared individual cognitive-behavioral therapy, group cognitive-behavioral therapy, and an educational-supportive psychotherapy that did not contain specific cognitive-behavioral therapy elements in treating patients with social anxiety disorder. They found that all three treatments produced significant reductions in symptoms and functional impairment, as well as improved social skills, with no differences between treatments. In another study of social anxiety disorder, Lipsitz et al. (2008) found that supportive psychotherapy and interpersonal therapy produced significant improvement from pretreatment to posttreatment, with neither therapy being superior to the other. However, Shear et al. (2001) reported that emotion-focused psychotherapy, a form of supportive psychotherapy, has low efficacy for the treatment of panic disorder. They compared emotion-focused psychotherapy with cognitive-behavioral treatment, imipramine, or pill placebo in a study involving 112 subjects.

Personality Disorder Studies

In a study comparing supportive with interpretive psychotherapy, Piper et al. (1998) found no outcome differences between the two treatments. Patients presented with anxiety or depressive disorders, and 60.4% of subjects had comorbid personality disorder. Hellerstein et al. (1998) compared brief supportive psychotherapy with short-term dynamic psychotherapy in treating patients with primarily Cluster C and not-otherwise-specified personality disorders, as well as comorbid Axis I disorders, such as depression or anxiety. The authors reported similar efficacy on measures of symptomatology, presenting complaints, and interpersonal functioning. These changes were found not only at termination but also at 6-month follow-up. In a substudy of the study by Hellerstein et al. (1998), the authors used the Inventory of Interpersonal Problems mapped to an interpersonal circumplex model and graphically demonstrated lasting positive change in interpersonal functioning in the subjects treated with supportive psychotherapy (Rosenthal et al. 1999; Winston et al. 2001).

Eating Disorder Studies

An evaluation of the efficacy of family-based treatment compared with supportive psychotherapy was undertaken by le Grange et al. (2007) for adolescent bulimia nervosa. Family-based treatment was found to have a clinical and statistical advantage over supportive psychotherapy.

Medical Disorder Studies

Mumford et al. (1982) reviewed controlled studies of supportive psychotherapy—including education about illness and treatments, cognitive-behavioral techniques, and ventilation and reassurance in a supportive relationship—in patients recovering from myocardial infarctions and surgery. The authors found that compared with patients receiving only typical medical care, patients receiving psychological intervention had better experiences with pain and increased patient compliance and speed of recovery, as well as fewer complications and fewer days in the hospital.

Conclusion

In this chapter, we have provided an overview of current efforts to evaluate the competence of residents engaged in various clinical tasks, and in particular supportive psychotherapy, as well as a summary of outcome research in supportive psychotherapy. We have presented a preliminary approach to evaluating psychiatry residents in supportive psychotherapy using an adaptation of the AADPRT list of supportive psychotherapy competencies. However, the process of evaluating competence is in an early phase of development and will require a great deal of reflection, planning, and study to achieve reliable and valid measurement systems.

The brief review of the efficacy of supportive psychotherapy indicates that supportive treatment appears to be useful across a broad spectrum of psychiatric and medical disorders. However, more research is needed to clarify the indications for supportive psychotherapy and how this treatment should be integrated with other psychotherapy approaches and treatment with medication.

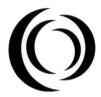

References

Accreditation Council for Graduate Medical Education: ACGME Program Requirements for Graduate Medical Education in Psychiatry. July 2007. Available at: www.acgme.org/acWebsite/downloads/RRC_progReq/400pr07012007.pdf. Accessed January 11, 2010.

Accreditation Council for Graduate Medical Education (ACGME) Outcomes Project: Toolbox of Assessment Methods, Version 1.1. September 2000. Available at: www.acgme.org/Outcome/assess/Toolbox.pdf. Accessed January 11, 2010.

Adshead G: Murmurs of discontent: treatment and treatability of personality disorder. Advances in Psychiatric Treatment 7:407–417, 2001

Aguilera DC, Messick J, Farrel LM: Crisis Intervention. St. Louis, MO, Mosby, 1970

Alcoholics Anonymous: The Story of How Many Thousands of Men and Women Have Recovered From Alcoholism, 3rd Edition. New York, Alcoholics Anonymous World Service, 1976, p 12

Alexander F, French TM: Psychoanalytic Psychotherapy. New York, Ronald Press, 1946

Alstrom JE, Nordlund CL, Persson G, et al: Effects of four treatment methods on social phobia patients not suitable for insight-oriented psychotherapy. Acta Psychiatr Scand 70:1–17, 1984

Alter CL: Palliative and supportive care of patients with pancreatic cancer. Semin Oncol 23:229–240, 1996

American Association of Directors of Psychiatric Residency Training Psychotherapy Task Force: Psychotherapy Competencies. Farmington, CT, American Association of Directors of Psychiatric Residency Training, 2000

American Psychiatric Association: Diagnostic and Statistical Manual of Mental Disorders, 4th Edition, Text Revision. Washington, DC, American Psychiatric Association, 2000

Appelbaum AH, Levy KN: Supportive psychotherapy for borderline patients: a psychoanalytic research perspective. Am J Psychoanal 62:201–202, 2002

Artiss KL: Human behavior under stress: from combat to social psychiatry. Mil Med 128:1011–1015, 1963

Balsam RM, Balsam A: Becoming a Psychotherapist: A Clinical Primer, 2nd Edition. Chicago, IL, University of Chicago Press, 1984

Bateman AW, Fonagy P: Effectiveness of psychotherapeutic treatment of personality disorder. Br J Psychiatry 177:138–143, 2000

Beck AT, Sokol L, Clark DA, et al: A crossover study of focused cognitive therapy for panic disorder. Am J Psychiatry 149:778–783, 1992

Beitman B, Yue D: Learning Psychotherapy: A Time-Efficient, Research-Based, and Outcome-Measured Training Program. New York, WW Norton, 1999

Bellack AS, Mueser KT: Psychosocial treatment for schizophrenia. Schizophr Bull 19:317–336, 1993

Bellak L: The schizophrenic syndrome: a further elaboration of the unified theory of schizophrenia, in Schizophrenia: A Review of the Syndrome. New York, Logos, 1958, pp 3–63

Beres D: Ego deviation and the concept of schizophrenia, in The Psychoanalytic Study of the Child, Vol 11. New York, International Universities Press, 1956, pp 164–235

Beutler LE, Moleiro C, Talebi H: Resistance in psychotherapy: what conclusions are supported by research. J Clin Psychol 58:207–217, 2002a

Beutler LE, Moleiro CM, Talebi H: Resistance, in Psychotherapy Relationships That Work: Therapist Contributions and Responsiveness to Patients. Edited by Norcross JC. London, Oxford University Press, 2002b, pp 129–143

Birmaher B, Brent DA, Kolko D, et al: Clinical outcome after short-term psychotherapy for adolescents with major depressive disorder. Arch Gen Psychiatry 57:29–36, 2000

Bond M, Banon E, Grenier M: Differential effects of interventions on the therapeutic alliance with patients with personality disorders. J Psychother Pract Res 7:301–318, 1998

Bordin E: The generalizability of the psycho-analytic concept of the working alliance. Psychotherapy: Theory, Research and Practice 16:252–260, 1979

Brent DA, Holder D, Kolko D, et al: A clinical psychotherapy trial for adolescent depression comparing cognitive, family, and supportive treatments. Arch Gen Psychiatry 54:877–885, 1997

Brill L: The treatment of drug abuse: evolution of a perspective. Am J Psychiatry 134:157–160, 1977

Bronheim HE, Fulop G, Kunkel EJ, et al: The Academy of Psychosomatic Medicine practice guidelines for psychiatric consultation in the general medical setting. The Academy of Psychosomatic Medicine. Psychosomatics 39:S8–S30, 1998

Bryant RA, Sackville T, Dang ST, et al: Treating acute stress disorder: an evaluation of cognitive behavior therapy and supportive counseling techniques. Am J Psychiatry 156:1780–1786, 1999

Buckley P: Supportive therapy: a neglected treatment. Psychiatr Ann 16:515–521, 1986

Busch KA, Fawcett J, Jacobs DG: Clinical correlates of inpatient suicide. J Clin Psychiatry 64:14–19, 2003

Caplan G: An Approach to Community Mental Health. New York, Grune & Stratton, 1961

Carey KB, Coco KM, Simons JS: Concurrent validity of clinicians' ratings of substance abuse among psychiatric outpatients. Psychiatr Serv 47:842–847, 1996

Clark DC, Fawcett J: A review of empirical risk factors for the evaluation of the suicidal patient, in The Assessment, Management, and Treatment of Suicide: Guidelines for Practice. Edited by Bongar B. New York, Oxford University Press, 1992, pp 16–48

Clarkin JF, Levy KN, Lenzenweger MF, et al: Evaluating three treatments for borderline personality disorder: a multiwave study. Am J Psychiatry 164:922–938, 2007

Classen C, Butler LD, Koopman C, et al: Supportive expressive group therapy and distress in patients with metastatic breast cancer: a randomized clinical intervention trial. Arch Gen Psychiatry 58:494–501, 2001

Clever SL, Tulsky JA: Dreaded conversations: moving beyond discomfort in patient-physician communication (editorial). J Gen Intern Med 17:893–894, 2002

Colby KM: A Primer for Psychotherapies. New York, The Ronald Press, 1951

Davanloo H: A method of short-term dynamic psychotherapy, in Short-Term Dynamic Psychotherapy. Edited by Davanloo H. Northvale, NJ, Jason Aronson, 1980, pp 43–71

de Jonghe F, Rijnierse P, Janssen R: The role of support in psychoanalysis. J Am Psychoanal Assoc 40:475–499, 1992

de Maat S, Dekker J, Schoevers R, et al: Short psychodynamic supportive psychotherapy, antidepressants, and their combination in the treatment of major depression: a mega-analysis based on three randomized clinical trials. Depress Anxiety 25:565–574, 2008

Dewald PA: The strategy of the therapeutic process, in Psychotherapy: A Dynamic Approach. New York, Basic Books, 1964, pp 95–108

Dewald PA: Psychotherapy: A Dynamic Approach, 2nd Edition. New York, Basic Books, 1971

Dewald PA: Principles of supportive psychotherapy. Am J Psychother 48:505–518, 1994

deWinstanley PA, Bjork RA: Successful lecturing: presenting information in ways that engage effective processing, in New Directions for Teaching and Learning. Edited by Halpern D, Hakel M. San Francisco, CA, Jossey-Bass, 2002, pp 19–31

Douglas CJ: Teaching supportive psychotherapy to psychiatric residents. Am J Psychiatry 165:445–452, 2008

Drake RE, Sederer LI: Inpatient psychosocial treatment of chronic schizophrenia: negative effects and current guidelines. Hosp Community Psychiatry 37:897–901, 1986

Drake RE, McHugo GJ, Noordsy DL: Treatment of alcoholism among schizophrenic outpatients: 4-year outcomes. Am J Psychiatry 150:328–329, 1993

Drake RE, Essock SM, Shaner A, et al: Implementing dual diagnosis services for clients with severe mental illness. Psychiatr Serv 52:469–476, 2001

Dunn C, Deroo L, Rivara FP: The use of brief interventions adapted from motivational interviewing across behavioral domains: a systematic review. Addiction 96:1725–1742, 2001

Elkin I: The NIMH Treatment of Depression Collaborative Research Program: where we began and where we are, in Handbook of Psychotherapy and Behavioral Change. Edited by Bergin AE, Garfield SL. New York, Wiley, 1994, pp 114–139

Elkin I, Shea MT, Watkins JT, et al: National Institute of Mental Health Treatment of Depression Collaborative Research Program. General effectiveness of treatments. Arch Gen Psychiatry 46:971–982, 1989

Epstein RM, Hundert EM: Defining and assessing professional competence. JAMA 287:226–235, 2002

Evans S, Fishman B, Spielman L, et al: Randomized trial of cognitive behavior therapy versus supportive psychotherapy for HIV-related peripheral neuropathic pain. Psychosomatics 44:44–50, 2003

Everly GS Jr, Mitchell JT: Assisting Individuals in Crisis: A Workbook. Ellicott City, MD, International Critical Incident Stress Foundation, 1998

Everly GS Jr, Mitchell JT: Critical Incident Stress Management (CISM): A New Era and Standard of Care in Crisis Intervention, 2nd Edition. Ellicott City, MD, Chevron Publishing, 1999

Fawcett J, Scheftner WA, Fogg L: Time-related predictors of suicide in major affective disorder. Am J Psychiatry 147:1189–1194, 1990

Fawcett J, Clark DC, Busch KA: Assessing and treating the patient at risk for suicide. Psychiatr Ann 23:244–255, 1993

Fernandez-Pol B, Bluestone H, Mizruchi MS: Inner-city substance abuse patterns: a study of psychiatric inpatients. Am J Drug Alcohol Abuse 14:41–50, 1988

Fischer DE, Halikas JA, Baker JW, et al: Frequency and patterns of drug abuse in psychiatric patients. Dis Nerv Syst 36:550–553, 1975

Foa EB: Trauma and women: course, predictors, and treatment. J Clin Psychiatry 58:25–28, 1997

Foa EB, Franklin ME: Psychotherapies for obsessive compulsive disorder: a review, in Obsessive Compulsive Disorder, 2nd Edition. Edited by Maj M, Sartorius N, Okasha A, et al. Chichester, England, Wiley, 2002, pp 93–115

Foa EB, Rothbaum BO, Riggs DS, et al: Treatment of posttraumatic stress disorder in rape victims: a comparison between cognitive-behavioral procedures and counseling. J Consult Clin Psychol 59:715–723, 1991

Fonagy P, Target M: Theoretical models of psychodynamic psychotherapy, in Textbook of Psychotherapeutic Treatments. Edited by Gabbard GO. Washington, DC, American Psychiatric Publishing, 2009, pp 3–42

Frank JD: General psychotherapy: the restoration of morale, in American Handbook of Psychiatry, Vol 5: Treatment, 2nd Edition. Edited by Freedman DX, Dyrud JE. New York, Basic Books, 1975, pp 117–132

Frank J, Frank J: Persuasion and Healing: A Comparison Study of Psychotherapy, 3rd Edition. Baltimore, MD, Johns Hopkins University Press, 1991

Freud S: The ego and the id (1923), in The Standard Edition of the Complete Psychological Works of Sigmund Freud, Vol 19. Edited by Strachey J. London, Hogarth Press, 1961, pp 12–66

Freud S: Inhibitions, symptoms and anxiety (1926), in The Standard Edition of the Complete Psychological Works of Sigmund Freud, Vol 20. Edited by Strachey J. London, Hogarth Press, 1959, pp 75–175

Friedman RS, Lister P: The current status of psychodynamic formulation. Psychiatry 50:126–141, 1987

Fudala PJ, Bridge TP, Herbert S, et al, and the Buprenorphine/Naloxone Collaborative Study Group: Office-based treatment of opiate addiction with a sublingual-tablet formulation of buprenorphine and naloxone. N Engl J Med 349:949–958, 2003

Fuller RK, Branchey L, Brightwell DR, et al: Disulfiram treatment of alcoholism: a Veterans Administration cooperative study. JAMA 256:1449–55, 1986

Gabbard GO: A contemporary psychoanalytic model of countertransference. J Clin Psychol 57:983–991, 2001

Gabbard GO: Long-Term Psychodynamic Psychotherapy: A Basic Text, 2nd Edition. Washington, DC, American Psychiatric Publishing, 2010

Galanter M, Castaneda R, Ferman J: Substance abuse among general psychiatric patients: place of presentation, diagnosis, and treatment. Am J Drug Alcohol Abuse 14:211–235, 1988

Gaston L: The concept of the alliance and its role in psychotherapy: theoretical and empirical considerations. Psychotherapy 27:143–153, 1990

Gelso CJ, Fassinger RE, Gomez MJ, et al: Countertransference reactions to lesbian clients: the role of homophobia, counselor gender, and countertransference management. J Couns Psychol 42:356–364, 1995

Gelso CJ, Latts MG, Gomez MJ, et al: Countertransference management and therapy outcome: an initial evaluation. J Clin Psychol 58:861–867, 2002

Gerstley L, McLellan AT, Alterman AI, et al: Ability to form an alliance with the therapist: a possible marker of prognosis for patients with antisocial personality disorder. Am J Psychiatry 146:508–512, 1989

Gill MM, Muslin HL: Early interpretation of transference. J Am Psychoanal Assoc 24:779–794, 1976

Glass A: Psychotherapy in the combat zone. Am J Psychiatry 110:725–731, 1954

Glover E: The therapeutic effect of inexact interpretation: a contribution to the theory of suggestion. Int J Psychoanal 12:397–411, 1931

Glynn SM, Marder SR, Liberman RP, et al: Supplementing clinic-based skills training with manual-based community support sessions: effects on social adjustment of patients with schizophrenia. Am J Psychiatry 159:829–837, 2002

Goldberg RL, Green SA: A learning-theory perspective of brief psychodynamic psychotherapy. Am J Psychotherapy 40:70–82, 1986

Goldman CR, Quinn FL: Effects of a patient education program in the treatment of schizophrenia. Hosp Community Psychiatry 39:282–286, 1988

Gorton GE: Psychodynamic approaches to the patient. Psychiatr Serv 51:1408–1409, 2000

Greenberg J: The analyst's participation: a new look. J Am Psychoanal Assoc 49:359–426, 2001

Greenson RR: The working alliance and the transference neurosis. Psychoanal Q 34:155–181, 1965

Greenson RR: The Technique and Practice of Psychoanalysis. New York, International Universities Press, 1967, pp 190–216

Gunderson JG, Frank AF, Katz HM, et al: Effects of psychotherapy in schizophrenia, II: comparative outcome of two forms of treatment. Schizophr Bull 10:564–598, 1984

Hartley DE, Strupp HH: The therapeutic alliance: its relationship to outcome in brief psychotherapy, in Empirical Studies of Psychoanalytical Theories, Vol 1. Edited by Masling J. Hillsdale, NJ, Analytic Press, 1983, pp 1–27

Hartmann H: Ego Psychology and the Problem of Adaptation (1939). Translated by Rapaport D. New York, International Universities Press, 1958

Hawton K: Assessment of suicide risk. Br J Psychiatry 150:145–154, 1987

Heinssen RK, Liberman RP, Kopelowicz A: Psychosocial skills training for schizophrenia: lessons from the laboratory. Schizophr Bull 26:21–46, 2000

Hellerstein DJ, Pinsker H, Rosenthal RN, et al: Supportive psychotherapy as the treatment model of choice. J Psychother Pract Res 3:300–306, 1994

Hellerstein DJ, Rosenthal RN, Miner CR: A prospective study of integrated outpatient treatment for substance-abusing schizophrenia patients. Am J Addict 4:33–42, 1995

Hellerstein DJ, Rosenthal RN, Pinsker H, et al: A randomized prospective study comparing supportive and dynamic therapies. Outcome and alliance. J Psychother Pract Res 7:261–271, 1998

Hellerstein DJ, Kocsis JH, Chapman D, et al: Double-blind comparison of sertraline, imipramine, and placebo in the treatment of dysthymia: effects on personality. Am J Psychiatry 157:1436–1444, 2000

Henry WP, Schacht TE, Strupp HH: Structural analysis of social behavior: application to a study of interpersonal process in differential psychotherapeutic outcome. J Consult Clin Psychol 54:27–31, 1986

Henry WP, Schacht TE, Strupp HH: Patient and therapist introject, interpersonal process, and differential psychotherapy outcome. J Consult Clin Psychol 58:768–774, 1990

Herbert JD, Gaudiano BA, Rheingold AA, et al: Cognitive behavior therapy for generalized social anxiety disorder in adolescents: a randomized controlled trial. J Anxiety Disord 23:167–177, 2009

Ho AP, Tsuang JW, Liberman RP, et al: Achieving effective treatment of patients with chronic psychotic illness and comorbid substance dependence. Am J Psychiatry 156:1765–1770, 1999

Hogarty GE, Kornblith SJ, Greenwald D, et al: Three-year trials of personal therapy among schizophrenia patients living with or independent of family, I: description of study and effects on relapse rates. Am J Psychiatry 154:1504–1513, 1997

Holmes J: Supportive psychotherapy. The search for positive meanings. Br J Psychiatry 167:439–445, 1995

Horowitz M, Marmar C: The therapeutic alliance with difficult patients, in Psychiatry Update: The American Psychiatric Association Annual Review, Vol 4. Edited by Hales RE, Frances AJ. Washington, DC, American Psychiatric Press, 1985, pp 573–585

Horowitz MJ, Marmar C, Weiss DS, et al: Brief psychotherapy of bereavement reactions. The relationship of process to outcome. Arch Gen Psychiatry 41:438–448, 1984

Horvath AO, Symonds BD: Relation between working alliance and outcome in psychotherapy: a meta-analysis. J Couns Psychol 38:139–149, 1991

Hunter J, Leszcz M, McLachlan SA, et al: Psychological stress response in breast cancer. Psychooncology 5:4–14, 1996

Imber SD, Pilkonis PA, Sotsky SM, et al: Mode-specific effects among three treatments for depression. J Consult Clin Psychol 58:352–359, 1990

James RK, Gilliland BE: Crisis Intervention Strategies, 4th Edition. Belmont, CA, Brooks/Cole Thomson Learning, 2001

Jellinek EM: Phases of alcohol addiction. Q J Stud Alcohol 13:673–684, 1952

Kates J, Rockland LH: Supportive psychotherapy of the schizophrenic patient. Am J Psychother 48:543–561, 1994

Kaufman ER: Countertransference and other mutually interactive aspects of psychotherapy with substance abusers. Am J Addict 1:185–202, 1992

Kaufman E, Reoux J: Guidelines for the successful psychotherapy of substance abusers. Am J Drug Alcohol Abuse 14:199–209, 1988

Keller DS, Carroll KM, Nick C, et al: Differential treatment response in alexithymic cocaine abusers: findings from a randomized clinical trial of psychotherapy and pharmacotherapy. Am J Addict 4:234–244, 1995

Kessler RC, McGonagle KA, Zhao S, et al: Lifetime and 12-month prevalence of DSM-III-R psychiatric disorders in the United States: results from the National Comorbidity Study. Arch Gen Psychiatry 51:8–19, 1994

Khantzian EJ: The self-medication hypothesis of addictive disorders: focus on heroin and cocaine dependence. Am J Psychiatry 142:189–198, 1985

Kiesler DJ: Therapist countertransference: in search of common themes and empirical referents. J Clin Psychol 57:1053–1063, 2001

Kleber HD: Pharmacologic treatments for heroin and cocaine dependence. Am J Addict 12 (suppl):S5–S18, 2003

Klein DF, Zitrin CM, Woerner MG, et al: Treatment of phobias, II: behavior therapy and supportive psychotherapy: are there any specific ingredients? Arch Gen Psychiatry 40:139–145, 1983

Kocsis JH, Gelenberg AJ, Rothbaum BO, et al: Cognitive behavioral analysis system of psychotherapy and brief supportive psychotherapy for augmentation of antidepressant nonresponse in chronic depression: the REVAMP Trial. Arch Gen Psychiatry 66:1178–1188, 2009

Kool S, Dekker J, Duijsens IJ, et al: Changes in personality pathology after pharmacotherapy and combined therapy for depressed patients. J Personal Disord 17:60–72, 2003

Koss M, Shiang J: Research on brief psychotherapy, in Handbook of Psychotherapy and Behavior Change. Edited by Bergin A, Garfield S. New York, John Wiley, 1994, pp 664–700

Lamberti JS, Herz MI: Psychotherapy, social skills training, and vocational rehabilitation in schizophrenia, in Contemporary Issues in the Treatment of Schizophrenia. Edited by Shriqui CL, Nasrallah HA. Washington, DC, American Psychiatric Press, 1995, pp 713–734

Lauriello J, Bustillo J, Keith SJ: A critical review of research on psychosocial treatment of schizophrenia. Biol Psychiatry 46:1409–1417, 1999

Lecomte T, Liberman RP, Wallace CJ: Identifying and using reinforcers to enhance the treatment of persons with serious mental illness. Psychiatr Serv 51:1312–1314, 2000

le Grange D, Crobsy RD, Rathouz PJ, et al: A randomized controlled comparison of family based treatment and supportive psychotherapy for adolescent bulimia nervosa. Arch Gen Psychiatry 64:1049–1056, 2007

Lehman AF, Herron D, Schwartz RP, et al: Rehabilitation for adults with severe mental illness and substance use disorders: a clinical trial. J Nerv Ment Dis 181:86–90, 1993

Lewis G, Appleby L: Personality disorder: the patients psychiatrists dislike. Br J Psychiatry 153:44–49, 1988

Liberman RP, Wallace CJ, Blackwell G, et al: Skills training versus psychosocial occupational therapy for persons with persistent schizophrenia. Am J Psychiatry 155:1087–1091, 1998

Lindemann E: Symptomatology and management of acute grief. Am J Psychiatry 101:141–148, 1944

Linehan MM: Cognitive-Behavioral Treatment of Borderline Personality Disorder. New York, Guilford, 1993

Linehan MM, Tutek DA, Heard HL, et al: Interpersonal outcome of cognitive behavioral treatment for chronically suicidal borderline patients. Am J Psychiatry 151:1771–1776, 1994

Lipsitz J, Gur M, Vermes D, et al: A randomized trial of interpersonal therapy versus supportive therapy for social anxiety disorder. Depress Anxiety 25:542–563, 2008

Luborsky L: Principles of Psychoanalytic Psychotherapy: A Manual for Support-ive-Expressive Treatment. New York, Basic Books, 1984

Luborsky L, Crits-Christoph P: Understanding Transference: The Core Conflict-ual Relationship Theme Method. New York, Basic Books, 1990

Luborsky L, Mark D: Short-term supportive-expressive psychoanalytic psycho-therapy, in Handbook of Short-Term Dynamic Psychotherapy. Edited by Crits-Christoph P, Barber JP. New York, Basic Books, 1991, pp 110–136

Maina G, Forner F, Bogetto F: Randomized controlled trial comparing brief dy-namic and supportive therapy with waiting list condition in minor depressive disorders. Psychother Psychosom 74:43–50, 2005

Malan DH: Individual Psychotherapy and the Science of Psychodynamics. Lon-don, Butterworth, 1979

Manring J, Beitman BD, Dewan MJ: Evaluating competence in psychotherapy. Paper presented at the annual meeting of the American Psychiatric Associa-tion, San Francisco, CA, May 2003

Markowitz JC, Klerman GL, Clougherty KF, et al: Individual psychotherapies for depressed HIV-positive patients. Am J Psychiatry 152:1504–1509, 1995

Marlatt GA, Gordon JR: Determinants of relapse: implications for the maintenance of behavior change, in Behavioral Medicine: Changing Health Lifestyles. Edited by Davidson PO, Davidson SM. New York, Brunner/Mazel, 1980, pp 410–452

Marlatt GA, Gordon JR: Relapse Prevention: Maintenance Strategies in the Treatment of Addictive Behaviors. New York, Guilford, 1985

Massie MJ, Holland JC: Depression and the cancer patient. J Clin Psychiatry 51 (suppl):12–19, 1990

McWilliams N: Psychoanalysis Psychotherapy: A Practitioner's Guide. New York, Guilford, 2004

Mellman LA, Beresin E: Psychotherapy competencies: development and imple-mentation. Academic Psychiatry 27:149–153, 2003

Menninger K: Theory of Psychoanalytic Technique. London, Imago, 1958

Messer SB: A psychodynamic perspective on resistance in psychotherapy: vive la résistance. J Clin Psychol 58:157–163, 2002

Mezirow J: On critical reflection. Adult Education Quarterly 48:185–198, 1998

Miller WR, Rollnick S: Motivational Interviewing: Preparing People to Change Addictive Behavior. New York, Guilford, 1991

Misch DA: Basic strategies of dynamic supportive therapy. J Psychother Pract Res 9:173–189, 2000

Mitchell JT, Everly GS Jr: Critical Incident Stress Debriefing (CISD): An Operations Manual for the Prevention of Traumatic Stress Among Emergency Service and Disaster Workers, 2nd Edition. Ellicott City, MD, Chevron Publishing, 1996

Mitchell JT, Everly GS Jr: Critical Incident Stress Management (CISM): Basic Group Crisis Intervention, 3rd Edition. Ellicott City, MD, International Crit-ical Incident Stress Foundation, 2003

Mitchell SA: Relational Concepts in Psychoanalysis: An Integration. Cambridge, MA, Harvard University Press, 1988

Mumford E, Schlesinger HJ, Glass CV: The effect of psychological intervention on recovery from surgery and heart attacks: an analysis of the literature. Am J Public Health 72:141–151, 1982

Novalis PN, Rojcewicz SJ, Peele R: Clinical Manual of Supportive Psychotherapy. Washington, DC, American Psychiatric Press, 1993

Nunberg H: The synthetic function of the ego. Int J Psychoanal 12:123–140, 1931

O'Malley SS, Jaffe AJ, Chang G, et al: Naltrexone and coping skills therapy for alcohol dependence: a controlled study. Arch Gen Psychiatry 49:881–887, 1992

Othmer E, Othmer S: The Clinical Interview Using DSM-IV, Vol 1. Washington, DC, American Psychiatric Press, 1994, pp 87–97

Palmer RL: Dialectical behavior therapy for borderline personality disorder. Advances in Psychiatric Treatment 8:10–16, 2002

Parad HJ, Parad LG: Crisis Intervention, Book 2: The Practitioner's Sourcebook for Brief Therapy. Milwaukee, WI, Family Service America, 1990

Parloff MB: Goals in psychotherapy: mediating and ultimate, in Goals of Psychotherapy. Edited by Mahrer AR. New York, Appleton-Century-Crofts, 1967, pp 5–19

Perry JC, Banon E, Ianni F: Effectiveness of psychotherapy for personality disorders. Am J Psychiatry 156:1312–1321, 1999

Perry S, Cooper AM, Michels R: The psychodynamic formulation: its purpose, structure, and clinical application. Am J Psychiatry 144:543–550, 1987

Persons JB: Cognitive Therapy in Practice: A Case Formulation Approach. New York, WW Norton, 1989

Persons JB: Case conceptualization in cognitive-behavior therapy, in Cognitive Therapies in Action: Evolving Innovative Practice. Edited by Kuehlwein KT, Rosen H. San Francisco, CA, Jossey-Bass, 1993, pp 33–53

Peselow ED, Sanfilipo MP, Fieve RR, et al: Personality traits during depression and after clinical recovery. Br J Psychiatry 164:349–354, 1994

Pine F: The interpretive moment. Variations on classical themes. Bull Menninger Clin 48:54–71, 1984

Pinsker H: A Primer of Supportive Psychotherapy. Hillsdale, NJ, Analytic Press, 1997

Pinsker H, Rosenthal RN: Beth Israel Medical Center Supportive Psychotherapy Manual (Social and Behavioral Sciences Documents, Vol 18, No 2). New York, Beth Israel Medical Center, 1988

Pinsker H, Rosenthal R, McCullough L: Dynamic supportive psychotherapy, in Handbook of Short-Term Dynamic Psychotherapy. Edited by Crits-Christoph P, Barber JP. New York, Basic Books, 1991, pp 220–247

Pinsker H, Hellerstein DJ, Rosenthal RN, et al: Supportive therapy, common factors and eclecticism. Paper presented at the annual meeting of the American Psychiatric Association, New York, May 1996

Pinsker H, Mellman L, Beresin E, et al: AADPRT Supportive Therapy Competencies. Lebanon, PA, American Association of Directors of Psychiatric Residency Training, November 2001

Piper WE, Joyce AS, McCallum M, et al: Interpretive and supportive forms of psychotherapy and patient personality variables. J Consult Clin Psychol 66:558–567, 1998

Pokorny AD: Prediction of suicide in psychiatric patients: report of a prospective study. Arch Gen Psychiatry 40:249–257, 1983

Pollack J, Flegenheimer W, Winston A: Brief adaptive psychotherapy, in Handbook of Short-Term Dynamic Psychotherapy. Edited by Crits-Christoph P, Barber JP. New York, Basic Books, 1991, pp 199–219

Posner K, Brent D, Lucas C, et al: Columbia-Suicide Severity Rating Scale (C-SSRS). New York, Columbia University/New York State Psychiatric Institute, 2009

Prochaska JO, DiClemente CC: The Transtheoretical Approach: Crossing Traditional Boundaries of Therapy. Homewood, IL, Dow Jones-Irwin, 1984

Psychopathology Committee of the Group for the Advancement of Psychiatry: Reexamination of therapist self-disclosure. Psychiatr Serv 52:1489–1493, 2001

Puryear DA: Helping People in Crisis. San Francisco, CA, Jossey-Bass, 1979

Quality Assurance Project: Treatment outlines for the management of the somatoform disorders. Aust N Z J Psychiatry 19:397–407, 1985

Rea MM, Strachan AM, Goldstein MJ, et al: Changes in coping style following individual and family treatment for schizophrenia. Br J Psychiatry 158:642–647, 1991

Regier DA, Farmer ME, Rae DS, et al: Comorbidity of mental disorders with alcohol and other drug abuse. Results from the Epidemiologic Catchment Area (ECA) study. JAMA 264:2511–2518, 1990

Renaud J, Brent DA, Baugher M, et al: Rapid response to psychosocial treatment for adolescent depression: a two-year follow-up. J Am Acad Child Adolesc Psychiatry 37:1184–1190, 1998

Richard ML, Liskow BI, Perry PJ: Recent psychostimulant use in hospitalized schizophrenics. J Clin Psychiatry 46:79–83, 1985

Robbins B: Under attack: devaluation and the challenge of tolerating the transference. J Psychother Pract Res 9:136–141, 2000

Roberts AR: An overview of crisis theory and crisis intervention, in Crisis Intervention Handbook. Edited by Roberts AR. New York, Oxford University Press, 2000, pp 3–30

Rockland LH: Supportive Therapy: A Psychodynamic Approach. New York, Basic Books, 1989

Rollnick S, Miller WR: What is motivational interviewing? Behavioral and Cognitive Psychotherapy 23:325–334, 1995

Rosenthal RN: Group treatments for schizophrenic substance abusers, in The Group Therapy of Substance Abuse. Edited by Brook DW, Spitz HI. New York, Haworth Medical Press, 2002, pp 329–351

Rosenthal RN: Techniques of individual supportive psychotherapy, in Textbook of Psychotherapeutic Treatments. Edited by Gabbard GO. Washington, DC, American Psychiatric Publishing, 2009, pp 417–445

Rosenthal RN, Westreich L: Treatment of persons with dual diagnoses of substance use disorder and other psychological problems, in Addictions: A Comprehensive Guidebook. Edited by McCrady GA, Epstein EE. New York, Oxford University Press, 1999, pp 439–476

Rosenthal RN, Muran JC, Pinsker H, et al: Interpersonal change in brief supportive psychotherapy. J Psychother Pract Res 8:55–63, 1999

Rosenthal RN, Miner CR, Sena P, et al: The therapeutic alliance in group treatments for substance abusers with schizophrenia, in Syllabus and Proceedings Summary, American Psychiatric Association Annual Meeting, Chicago, IL, May 14–19, 2000, Washington, DC, American Psychiatric Association

Rosenzweig S: Some implicit common factors in diverse methods of psychotherapy. Am J Orthopsychiatry 6:412–415, 1936

Rounsaville BJ, Carroll KM: Individual psychotherapy, in Principles of Addiction Medicine. Edited by Graham AW, Schultz TK. Chevy Chase, MD, American Society of Addiction Medicine, 1998, pp 631–652

Safran JD, Muran JC: Negotiating the Therapeutic Alliance: A Relational Treatment Guide. New York, Guilford, 2000, pp 6–12

Salmon TW: War neuroses and their lesson. New York Medical Journal 59:993–994, 1919

Sampson H, Weiss J: Testing hypotheses: the approach of the Mount Zion Psychotherapy Research Group, in The Psychotherapeutic Process: A Research Handbook. Edited by Greenberg LS, Pinsof WM. New York, Guilford, 1986, pp 591–613

Sandoval J: Crisis counseling: conceptualizations and genetic principles. School Psych Rev 14:257–265, 1985

Shear KM, Houck P, Greeno C, et al: Emotion-focused psychotherapy for patients with panic disorder. Am J Psychiatry 158:1993–1998, 2001

Sifneos PE: The prevalence of 'alexithymic' characteristics in psychosomatic patients. Psychother Psychosom 22:255–262, 1973

Sifneos PE: Problems of psychotherapy of patients with alexithymic characteristics and physical disease. Psychother Psychosom 26:65–70, 1975

Simon JC: Criteria for therapist self-disclosure. Am J Psychother 42:404–415, 1988

Skaikeu KA: Crisis Intervention. Boston, Allyn & Bacon, 1990

Smith TE, Hull JW, Goodman M, et al: The relative influences of symptoms, insight, and neurocognition on social adjustment in schizophrenia and schizoaffective disorder. J Nerv Ment Dis 187:102–108, 1999

Spiegel D, Classen C: Acute stress disorders, in Treatments of Psychiatric Disorders, 2nd Edition. Edited by Gabbard GO. Washington, DC, American Psychiatric Press, 1995, pp 1521–1536

Stanton AH, Gunderson JG, Knapp PH, et al: Effects of psychotherapy in schizophrenia, I: design and implementation of a controlled study. Schizophr Bull 10:520–563, 1984

Thomas EM, Weiss SM: Nonpharmacological interventions with chronic cancer pain in adults. Cancer Control 7:157–164, 2000

Thompson LW, Gallagher D: Depression and its treatment. Aging (Milano) 348:14–18, 1985

Tompkins MA: Cognitive-behavioral case formulation: the case of Jim. Journal of Psychotherapy Integration 6:97–105, 1996

Ursano RJ, Silberman EK: Psychoanalysis, psychoanalytic psychotherapy, and supportive psychotherapy, in The American Psychiatric Press Textbook of Psychiatry, 3rd Edition. Edited by Hales RE, Yudofsky SC, Talbott JA. Washington, DC, 1999, pp 1157–1183

Vaillant GE: Adaptation to Life. Boston, MA, Little, Brown, 1977

Vaillant GE (ed): Empirical Studies of Ego Mechanisms of Defense. Washington, DC, American Psychiatric Press, 1986

van Emmerik AAP, Kamphuis JH, Hulsbosch AM, et al: Single session debriefing after psychological trauma: a meta-analysis. Lancet 360:766–771, 2002

Vaughn CE, Leff JP: The influence of family and social factors on the course of psychiatric illness: a comparison of schizophrenic and depressed neurotic patients. Br J Psychiatry 129:125–137, 1976

Viederman M: A model for interpretive supportive dynamic psychotherapy. Psychiatry 71:349–358, 2008

Volpicelli JR, Alterman AI, Hayashida M, et al: Naltrexone in the treatment of alcohol dependence. Arch Gen Psychiatry 49:876–880, 1992

Wachtel P: Therapeutic Communication: Principles and Effective Practice. New York, Guilford, 1993

Wallerstein RS: Forty-Two Lives in Treatment: A Study of Psychoanalysis and Psychotherapy. New York, Guilford, 1986

Wallerstein RS: The psychotherapy research project of the Menninger Foundation: an overview. J Consult Clin Psychol 57:195–205, 1989

Walsh BT, Wilson GT, Loeb K, et al: Medication and psychotherapy in the treatment of bulimia nervosa. Am J Psychiatry 154:523–531, 1997

Waltz J, Addis ME, Koerner K, et al: Testing the integrity of a psychotherapy protocol: assessment of adherence and competence. J Consult Clin Psychol 61:620–630, 1993

Werman DS: The Practice of Supportive Psychotherapy. New York, Brunner/Mazel, 1984

Westerman MA, Foote JP, Winston A: Change in coordination across phases of psychotherapy and outcome: two mechanisms for the role played by patient's contribution to the alliance. J Consult Clin Psychol 24:190–195, 1995

Wilhelm S, Deckersbach T, Coffey B, et al: Habit reversal versus supportive psychotherapy for Tourette's disorder: a randomized controlled trial. Am J Psychiatry 160:1175–1177, 2003

Wilkinson CB, Vera E: Management and treatment of disaster victims. Psychiatr Ann 15:174–184, 1985

Winnicott DW: The Maturational Process and the Facilitating Environment: Studies in the Theory of Emotional Development. London, Hogarth Press, 1965

Winston A, Winston B: Handbook of Integrated Short-Term Psychotherapy. Washington, DC, American Psychiatric Publishing, 2002

Winston A, Pinsker H, McCullough L: A review of supportive psychotherapy. Hosp Community Psychiatry 37:1105–1114, 1986

Winston A, Rosenthal RN, Muran JC: Supportive psychotherapy, in Handbook of Personality Disorders: Theory, Research, and Treatment. Edited by Livesley WJ. New York, Guilford, 2001, pp 344–358

Woody GE, McLellan AT, Luborsky L, et al: Sociopathy and psychotherapy outcome. Arch Gen Psychiatry 42:1081–1086, 1985

Zetzel ER: Current concepts of transference. Int J Psychoanal 37:369–376, 1956

Ziedonis D, Fisher W: Motivation-based assessment and treatment of substance abuse in patients with schizophrenia. Directions in Psychiatry 16:1–7, 1996

Ziedonis D, Trudeau K: Motivation to quit using substances among individuals with schizophrenia: implications for a motivation-based treatment model. Schizophr Bull 23:229–238, 1997

Zitrin CM, Klein DF, Woerner MG, et al: Behavior therapy, supportive psychotherapy, imipramine, and phobias. Arch Gen Psychiatry 35:307–316, 1978

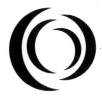

Index

*Page numbers printed in **boldface** type refer to tables or figures.*